The Hidden Hormone Solution

Discover the Secret to Health and Vitality at Any Age

The Hidden Hormone Solution

Discover the Secret to Health and
Vitality at Any Age

By Trevor Botts, DC

ISBN: 978-1-945446-02-3

YouSpeakIt
PUBLISHING
The Easy Way
to Get Your Book
Done Right ™

www.YouSpeakItPublishing.com

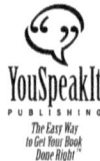

Dedication

This book is dedicated to the hope for a healthier, happier community.

Acknowledgments

Thank you to my family—my wife Mandy, my kids, parents, grandparents, and siblings—the big "why" in my life.

Thank you to all our practice members at Inspire Wellness Center who uplift me every day with their experiences of transformation and healing.

Thank you to Min Kwon for helping with the research that supports this book.

Thank you to Lindsey Keown for being a great wellness concierge to our practice members.

Thank you to Dr. Charles Webb, Cesar Torres, and the entire staff at Freedom Practice Coaching for helping me create a revolutionary wellness practice.

Thank you to the teachers, mentors, and coaches who help me be a better practitioner.

Thank you, God, for life and healing.

Foreword

Do any of these conditions sound familiar to you?

- Depressed
- Diabetic
- Overweight in spite of repeated attempts to lose weight
- Pain in the knees, feet, back, hands
- Tired all the time but unable to sleep well at night

That was the state of my health when I met Dr. Trevor Botts in August 2015.

As I listened to the information he shared — all of which is contained in this book — I began to hope that there was an answer to *why* I felt as I did; why I had tried and failed at diets for more than forty years; why I woke up every day feeling old.

Over the past eighteen months, I've had the pleasure of learning from and working with Dr. Botts to address my discomfort. I learned that each of these symptoms was actually a part of a deeper problem. And while traditional medicine strives to treat the symptoms with surgery or medicine, Dr. Botts' approach goes to the root cause.

With his professional insight and caring perspective, we have uncovered a myriad of underlying, interwoven reasons for my issues. I am certain I could never have done this without his help.

As the cause of each of my symptoms was revealed and addressed through nutrition and lifestyle changes, the problems disappeared:

- I have lost one hundred pounds.
- I am no longer diabetic.
- I don't hurt anymore, regardless of my activity level.
- My depression is gone! I wake up happy every morning, thankful that I found Dr. Botts.

I am convinced that no matter how many other solutions I might have tried, nothing could have served me as well as Dr. Botts' expert guidance. His approach made sense and was easy to adopt. And it all started with the information in this book.

You will be tempted to jump to the chapter that addresses your most pressing issue. Go ahead and start there. But be sure you go back to the beginning so that you understand the context of your current lifestyle choices. It will all finally make sense and get you started on the correct path to the relief of your symptoms and a lifetime of better health.

I know that, with this book in hand, you will find the beginning of your journey to wellness.

Jeanette S. Cates, PhD
Author, JeanettesJourney.com
Austin, Texas
March 2016

Table of Contents

Introduction

Have you ever noticed how some people seem to age more gracefully than others?

You may notice that some of your neighbors, friends, or family members appear to thrive in their golden years. One great example of agelessness is Jack LaLanne, the fitness guru. He had a long-running exercise program, *The Jack LaLanne Show,* on television and was the picture of health and vitality throughout his life. He helped a lot of people put together great fitness routines for themselves, and later in life became an advocate for healthy eating and nutrition.

I had the privilege of seeing Jack LaLanne on his ninety-fourth birthday. I was in school at the time, and he was invited to a large convention of students and doctors. It was a great celebration: the center was decked with birthday decorations and balloons, and even the Dallas Cowboy Cheerleaders were on hand to welcome LaLanne.

When Jack was introduced, he came slowly out onto the stage, bent over and leaning on a cane. The room fell silent, and it was clear that everyone was shocked to see this man, known for his incredible strength and health, now reduced to frailty and falling apart.

He hobbled to the center of the stage, looked up at us, and very weakly said into the microphone, "Thank you for coming out and celebrating with me."

Then LaLanne tossed his cane off to the side, jumped up in the air, and called out, "How's everybody doing?"

He started marching around the stage with vigor, practically doing backflips across the stage. It was incredible to be so limber at his age. All of the students and doctors erupted into wild applause for this man who was such a great example of health—and a great comedian, too.

For those of you who think that you are too old to be proactive and start to turn around years of stress and deteriorating health, just remember that at the age of seventy, Jack LaLanne swam Long Beach Harbor against strong winds, handcuffed and shackled, while towing seventy rowboats (one for each year of his life), one of which had several people sitting in it, for one full mile.

If LaLanne did that at the age of seventy, I believe that any motivated individual at any age can start to turn around their health.

On the flip side, why is it that some people just seem to deteriorate as they age, and their health seems gets worse and worse as time goes on?

In fact, with improvements in healthcare, although it is true that we are living longer, it seems to me that we're actually just *dying* longer.

The underlying cause for most of the ill health that we experience is *stress*. It is well understood that stress, in one form or another, has negative effects on our well-being:

- Physical stress or trauma, such as experiencing a car accident

- Chemical stress from pollutants in the air and toxins in our food

- Emotional stress; for example, caused by an angry coworker or rush-hour traffic

- Stress from infectious agents such as bacteria and viruses

We are all exposed to physical, chemical, and emotional stressors. Jack LaLanne, during his wonderful life, was exposed to just as many (if not more) stressors as anybody else. Yet some people seem to manage that stress; they stay healthy while others get sick.

Why is that?

The answer is that it's not the stressors — it's the person. It's your ability, or inability, to adapt to stressors that makes or breaks your health.

If you want to get a good idea of the negative impact that stress can have on your health, and how this can send you down a path to early disease, I want you to look back with me at a young, energetic, and enthusiastic Trevor Botts, who was in school for many years preparing to be a doctor who would educate his community about health and wellness.

While I was going through school, I was under incredible amounts of stress, as you can imagine:

- Countless long days and long nights

- A lot of studying

- A lot of sitting in class, not being active, not getting outdoors

- A lot of poor eating, or not eating at all

- Skipping meals because of a strenuous school schedule

When I finished my doctorate program in 2011 at the age of twenty-nine, I was actually in the worst health of my life.

Ironic, isn't it?

A doctor who was ready to go out and *heal the world* was actually in the worst health of his life:

- I came out of school forty pounds heavier than I am today and prediabetic.

- I was under incredible amounts of stress as I started my clinical work.

- I was having heart palpitations.

- I wasn't sleeping at night.

- I was a brand-new father, with all the stresses of supporting my family.

In pursuit of my health degree, I had ultimately neglected my own health. Very early on I realized that if I were going to be able to help anyone turn around *their* poor health, I had to first do it for myself.

People often ask me, "How did you, as a chiropractor, end up doing something in health that is not traditional chiropractic?"

The answer is, I always knew I wanted to help people be healthy, so I started down a premed path in college. But I noticed that our medical system—while wonderful at saving lives in an emergency—fails to help people achieve true health and vitality. I learned that drugs would never be able to replace healthy nutrition and lifestyle in improving health. I learned that if I really want to help people with *health* rather than *sickness,* I would need to find a different path.

I found that chiropractic has a strong philosophy of holistic (whole person) health and a respect and appreciation for the innate ability of the body to heal. So, I decided that would be the best place for me to receive my doctorate-level training. After school, it was through working on my own health concerns and those of my family that I found the world of functional wellness. It is a growing branch of health that can be practiced by any health practitioner who pursues the required advanced training. I realized that I could have an even greater impact on the health and well-being of my clients by *teaching* them how to take care of their own health.

I don't write this book as a doctor claiming to have a treatment, a magic pill, or a quick fix for any type of disease. In fact, there really is no doctor who can cure you of anything. Ultimately, it is *you* and your body who have to do the healing.

It is my hope for you that through reading this book you will become motivated and inspired to do the same thing that I did: take control of your own health.

Don't let anybody tell you that your health problem is just the genetic hand of cards that you were dealt, and you simply have to live with it. Be wary of anyone telling you that you have to just take pills to get over your illness. The body has an incredible ability to heal, if we will simply understand why things aren't working, and then provide the appropriate support for it to heal.

Why do you think the United States is one of the sickest countries in the world?

Well, the simple answer is that the American lifestyle creates an environment that causes stress to the body, in many different ways. This accumulation of stress creates the state of *dis-ease* in which the body is no longer able to adapt to stressors. That is when the body becomes sick.

The signs and symptoms of a body failing to adapt can be seen early on, long before a true disease process has taken hold. Often, these early signs of stress affect the delicate balance of hormones in the body. By understanding how these hormones function, we can identify what a person with an underlying hormone imbalance looks like and feels like. More important, we can learn to take action early on, before a lifelong disease has developed, and we can effectively reverse the effects of years of stress on the body.

In this book, I inform you about the four most common hormone imbalances that occur as the body loses its ability to adapt to stress. I help you identify if you might be developing one of these hormone problems, and then tell you what you can do about it.

Please understand, our hormone systems are incredibly complex, and I could fill volumes exploring them. This book is meant as only an introduction. Also, my intention is not to simply create a how-to manual on addressing hormone dysfunction. As you will see, these issues will oftentimes require a personalized level of testing and care.

Furthermore, I always recommend that anyone dealing with a health issue be guided appropriately by a qualified healthcare professional.

I do, however, offer general guidelines for successful health management.

Think of this book as more of a *why-to* manual: Why it is important for you to understand these hormone systems, the effect that stress has on our bodies, and how you can go about finding the right help.

Before we jump into covering these different hormone systems, we first need to talk about how we got into this mess. Let's begin with our country's health crisis and the way that we have managed our health up until now.

CHAPTER
ONE

America's Health Crisis

*Insanity: Doing the same thing over and over
again and expecting different results.*
~ Albert Einstein

THE DEFINITION OF INSANITY

Our country spends more on health expenses than any
other nation, yet remains one of the sickest in the world.

I don't need to say much to convince anyone that the
health of our nation's people is in a crisis. If you look
around, you're going to see that most people in the
United States are fat, sick, and generally depressed. It
seems that the more we try to correct these problems
with our current way of dealing with health issues,
the worse they become. We spend twice as much on
healthcare as any other country in the world, yet our life
expectancy isn't among even the top twenty countries
(WHO, 2015). Americans take more medications than
the people in any other country. The list of the meds we
take continues to grow year after year, yet the rate of all
major illnesses in the United States continues to climb.

This current crisis in our country has led to some healthcare professionals actually calling our *health-care* system a *disease-management* system, meaning that rather than offering any type of resolution for health concerns, it simply manages the disease process until the person eventually loses their independence and quality of life.

If It's Not Working Now, When Will It?

I meet a lot of people who are very frustrated with their health. They're not sure what they should be doing, yet they find that what they are currently doing doesn't seem to be working, whether it's a prescription medication or a diet fad or supplement trend or workout routine.

I always ask the following questions:

- If what you're doing right now isn't working, at what point do you expect that it will finally start to kick in?

- If you take thyroid hormones and they didn't seem to be working yesterday, do you expect them to suddenly start working today?

- If you take metformin and insulin for diabetes, at what point do you expect that the drug will finally cure you?

- If you're on a cholesterol medication, at what point do you expect that you'll finally be able to stop taking it, if all the medication has done is to artificially lower your cholesterol values?

- If what you're doing right now isn't working, is it fair to say that you probably need to be doing something different?

I could mention all of the major degenerative diseases that people suffer from today, and point out that what most people are doing to manage their health isn't working, and yet somehow patients still expect that they will experience a cure someday. Einstein would call these patients insane.

If our current medical system isn't working, is it reasonable to say that you probably also need to look for a different system in order to find the health that you've been looking for and to finally resolve your health concerns?

If I'm going to do anything different for you, in terms of the recommendations that I make — either through this book or through the information that I share with you — then I also need to be a different kind of a doctor.

This is why I am not a traditional allopathic doctor. *Allopathic* is a term meaning medicine that depends on mainstream interventions, either physical or through the use of drugs, to treat symptoms instead of treating the whole person. I don't treat disease or symptoms with drugs or surgery; instead, I take the word *doctor* back to its Latin root, which means "teacher."

Decide to Break Free

The decision is yours: either continue down this same broken path or take control of your own health and break free of the inevitable sickness that awaits most Americans as they age.

One of my mentors refers to America's sickness-care system as a conveyor belt to poor health. What he means by this is that, if we don't choose to take control of our own health, then the system will manage it for us. If you do allow that system to manage your health, then it is very similar to simply riding down a conveyor belt.

Along that ride, you will inevitably be handed prescription medications and pills that manage your disease and its symptoms, but do not actually offer any type of resolution or cure of the underlying causes. These medications will not actually support any healing processes in the body. And that list of pills, for many individuals, will get longer and longer as the ride progresses. At the end of that ride, there is ultimately only one destination for everyone who chooses not to be proactive toward their health.

Ultimately, it ends in:

- A loss of independence
- A loss of quality of life
- Ultimately, a loss of life

That is why it is on your shoulders to make that decision.

I can tell you from personal experience that this conveyor belt will wreak havoc on a person's life if it is allowed to manage their health. Let me tell you about a gentleman I knew when I was growing up. His name was Herb. He played trumpet in local community bands, and as a young trumpeter I looked up to him. He was an Eagle Scout, and I was a Scout as well. He was a wonderful mentor for me.

Like many Americans, Herb was diagnosed with a number of health concerns:

- Diabetes
- High blood pressure
- High cholesterol

Herb had been taught that our current system could manage his illness, so he took the medications that were prescribed for him, as many individuals do. For several decades, he really felt fine; he didn't feel like anything was broken or not working, even though the disease was beginning to progress internally.

As I was going though my health training, I would check in with Herb and see how he was doing. I would share with him information about some of the alternative things that we were learning in school — about being proactive toward our health — and Herb was very impressed by all of this, but for one reason or another it didn't quite fit with what he was willing to do for himself. He didn't make any significant lifestyle changes, and slowly, over time, his health continued to deteriorate.

Over time, Herb noticed several changes in his health:

- He was no longer able to walk around the lake with his wife and friends.

- He felt weaker, winded, and fatigued.

- He developed some body aches and pains as his diabetes continued to progress.

- He experienced the typical numbness, tingling, and burning sensations caused by diabetes, especially in his legs and feet.

Herb's wife once found him in their driveway, sweeping away the leaves in freezing-cold weather while wearing only his slippers, not aware of the cold because he couldn't feel his feet anymore. Eventually he developed shingles and a low-back disc herniation. His blood pressure continued to worsen, and he ended up more or less confined to his bed for long periods of time.

Herb woke up one day and realized he had fallen off the end of the allopathic medical conveyor belt: He had lost his independence and quality of life. It's heartbreaking to see someone whom you love go through something like this . . . especially when he's your grandfather.

It was especially difficult for me to watch my grandfather, Herb, in declining health because I was learning about different ways that his condition could be supported. I was learning about how to help people break free of the so-called healthcare system and create a better life — and better health — for themselves. We hope that my grandfather will be with us for many more years to come. But it has become a huge challenge for our family, as it has for many people who need to help their loved ones in failing health.

Ultimately, my goal for you as you read through this book is to help you finally *stop the insanity* — and take control of your health.

OUR CURRENT HEALTHCARE SYSTEM CAN-NOT TREAT MOST PREVALENT DISEASES

Ninety percent of diseases prevalent today are not treatable with orthodox medical procedures.
~ World Health Organization

Most Diseases Are Chronic, Resulting From Lifestyle Choices

Hopefully this statistic is disturbing to you: 90 percent of the diseases that are killing most of us today cannot be cured within our current medical system.

That's what the World Health Organization is reporting. When you think about it, it actually makes a lot of sense, because 90 percent of diseases are chronic and based on lifestyle. Most of the illnesses that people suffer from today are slow, degenerative processes, and lifestyle is either a cause or a contributing factor. Our medical system is designed to treat only crises and acute illnesses, such as broken bones, wounds, infections, and emergency surgery such as open-heart surgery, and it excels in these fields, but not in chronic illness.

For example, consider type 2 diabetes, a chronic condition, and the story about my grandfather, Herb. Type 2 diabetes is completely preventable and controllable through proper lifestyle choices.

Unfortunately, 25 percent of the population over the age of sixty-five in our country is diabetic, and about a third of these people don't even know that they suffer from this condition.

Sadly, about 50 percent of children born after the year 2000 are expected to become diabetic within their lifetimes, and it is expected that diabetes alone will bankrupt our entire healthcare system. Just the other day, I met a two-year-old boy who weighs almost forty pounds. He weighs as much as a healthy five- or six-year-old and he's on the road toward diabetes at the age of two, and all of this is completely preventable (Centers for Disease Control, 2014).

The 10 Percent Who Can Be Treated

Let's back up for a moment and give credit where credit is due. Who exactly represents the 10 percent who *can* be successfully treated within our current medical system? I've already touched on it briefly: It's those people who need crisis intervention or have an emergency. If you need some type of drug or surgery *right now* in order to save your life, be glad that our healthcare system is ready for you.

Please understand: I'm not bashing our medical system, or any of our medical doctors. When it comes to saving your life, we really, truly have the best physicians to care for you. If I ever need open-heart surgery, you better believe I'm going to tell them to crack my chest open to get it done. If you need antibiotics right now, or you might lose your leg to infection, I'm sure you will be glad that they are readily available.

The problem is that our health profile as a nation has changed so much within only the past few decades. It's not infections, acute illnesses, and emergency health crises that are killing us. These are actually being fairly well managed. What are becoming more and more problematic are lifestyle-based chronic diseases. They are becoming a true epidemic. They simply *cannot* be successfully treated or managed through this allopathic drug-and-surgery type of approach.

For example, if your house is on fire—it's burning to the ground and you're scrambling to get all of your loved ones and valuables out of the house as quickly as you can—who are you going to call?

Obviously, you will call the fire department, and you're going to ask them to do anything that is necessary in order to save as much of the house as possible.

The fire department will come with ladders and hoses and axes. They'll kick in the doors and the windows. They actually cause a lot of destruction to your house— what remains will be soaked with water from the hoses—but they're doing this because they are seeking to put out every single flame and save the integrity of your home. You're going to be very grateful to them for offering this service.

This is similar to the emergency care that our medical system can offer when you are in a crisis.

But what are you going to do when the crisis is over and you need to start rebuilding?

In the case of the fire, it would be silly to call the same firefighters and ask them to come back and start to rebuild your home, because that's not what they're trained for; it's not their specialty. You need a contractor with a team of carpenters and electricians and plumbers to fix your house. It's a similar situation when it comes to our health.

When it comes to saving your life, we truly have the best physicians and surgeons to do exactly that. But once the emergency is over, you need to have the appropriate help in order to start to rebuild your health. Unfortunately, our system simply doesn't offer this.

If you're part of that 10 percent—dealing with an acute medical emergency—be glad you are getting the help you need.

For the 90 percent of us who are dealing with chronic diseases, the last thing you want to do is to be looking for help from our emergency-focused system.

They will say, "Well, we can't help you with that, but here's some medication to manage your symptoms."

Then they'll set you on that conveyor belt until your health does become a crisis, when they can offer you all the wonderful drugs and surgery available.

Reality Check: What Does Our Insurance Actually Pay For?

We need to talk about insurance, because in my opinion, this is a big part of our nation's health crisis. We have allowed insurance to be a crutch for far too long. It has put many people into their graves prematurely, because we have been taught and we believe that someone else is going to take care of us, and someone else is going to pay to manage our health. In fact, there are even groups that claim that all of our health problems would be solved if everyone had medical insurance.

But here's the reality check: Does your life insurance do anything to protect your life?

Well, no.

When does it pay out?

When you're dead. We should really call it *death insurance*.

What about your health insurance? Does it actually do anything to protect or enhance your health?

No, because it pays out only when you're sick. And when you are sick, as already discussed, the only two things that our medical system can offer you are drugs and surgery.

I mentioned before that 90 percent of diseases cannot be treated with our orthodox medical procedures.

But at the same time, isn't it true that our health insurance is designed to pay only for orthodox medical procedures?

Insurance companies are often the ones that get to decide what is considered the correct medicine for a given health problem. If we follow this reasoning to its logical conclusion, this means that your insurance pays for what *doesn't* work 90 percent of the time. And we wonder why, as a country, we continue to be so sick.

I have health insurance. I have never used it and I never plan on using it. But I think it's a good idea to have insurance in the event of a health crisis. After all, that's what insurance is designed for. But I understand that paying my premium is not an investment toward my health — instead, it is an expense, because I never expect to get back any of the money I dump into it.

If I ever do use that insurance, it will mean that I have probably fallen into an emergency or crisis, or I won the jackpot on some type of disease that's going to require an expensive procedure. That is the only way my insurance will ever pay out more than I pay in. But I don't know anyone who would really want to win that lottery. I think we would all rather simply have our health.

True health "insurance" doesn't come from paying a premium; it comes from investing a little time, effort, and money into a healthy lifestyle. Invest in your health now, or pay for it later.

WHAT IS THE SOLUTION TO OUR HEALTH CRISIS?

I've covered thus far why our country is in the big mess that it's in. I think it's only fair that I take a moment to describe to you what the solution to this crisis really is.

What Is Functional Wellness?

Where traditional medicine tends to simply identify or diagnose a disease or a symptom and then manage it with drugs, *functional wellness* goes deeper, to a more foundational level, and asks the question, "Why?"

Why are things not working for this person?

Why is this organ system not functioning?

Why is this person's body not able to heal?

Once we've determined the underlying cause of dysfunction, rather than simply mask it or cover it up with drugs and medications, we seek to teach the person and educate them about what it is that they can be doing to take control of their health. Through this approach, we support the body's innate ability to heal itself. It can be a very rewarding approach, but obviously it does require that the person be accountable and proactive.

An "Inspire Wellness" Experience

From the first day I walked into the Inspire Wellness Center, I felt welcome and cared for, and I couldn't be happier with my results! I highly recommend Dr. Botts to all my friends and family now. I have yet to find another doctor who cares about a person's well-being as much as he does.

~ Toni T.
Austin, Texas

The Wilting Plant

In many ways, you already want to think like a functional wellness practitioner — you just don't know it yet. Let me prove it to you. Imagine that you see a wilting plant in your home.

What's the very first thing that you would think of?

Water, of course, and then what?

Sunlight.

Then maybe nutrients in the soil.

What is interesting is that the very first thing that you probably decided to do wasn't to immediately put some pesticides or fungicides or some type of a chemical on this plant.

When it comes to something as simple and beautiful as a plant, we seem to understand that there are basic foundational principles that need to be in place in order for that plant to thrive. We don't immediately assume that it requires a chemical intervention in order to heal.

Could you simply paint the leaves green, which might make the plant look a little bit better?

Well, of course you could. But meanwhile, it's still dying on the inside.

How many people around you that you know and care about are painting their leaves green every single day, in the form of medications and pills and chemicals that cover up their problems?

Meanwhile, they're still suffering on the inside.

The Wilting Human

If we see a wilting human — someone who is struggling and in pain — typically the very first questions that practitioners in the allopathic medical system will ask are, "What is your diagnosis? What condition do you have?"

They ask these questions so that they can then decide what drugs or surgery to give to you. It's interesting that when it comes to our own health, we seem to jump right over all of the simple solutions — water, sunlight, nutrients — that we naturally think about when we are treating a wilting plant.

Our current medical system considers, "What type of intervention can we impose on this person in order to manage their health?" instead of examining how to support your ability to heal.

The reason that we have a tendency to think this way about our own health is because we have been conditioned to believe that our health will come from pills. This is no accident. Pharmaceutical companies spend billions of dollars every year to train us to think this way. Just turn on the TV and every other commercial is advertising some type of a drug for some type of symptom.

At the end, the announcer always says, "Ask your doctor about this particular drug."

These companies are actually turning us into their own (unpaid) pharmaceutical sales reps, so that we will go to our doctors and ask them to put us on a specific medication. The doctor will check your diagnosis, and then they'll check the list of allowed medications. If they see that whatever you're asking for is on the approved list, they'll go ahead and write that script for you. This is, again, no mistake. These drug companies know what they're doing, and they want to control your health through this medication model.

The tragedy is that, because most diseases are chronic and degenerative, they are not treatable with this medication approach.

That means prescription drugs are prescribed for life for conditions such as:

- Diabetes
- Autoimmune disorders
- High cholesterol
- Heart disease

These all require prescription drugs for life. If you haven't been told when you get to go off this drug, it means that they expect you to take it for your lifetime. If you stop taking that drug, and things go right back to the way that they were before, then that means that the medication is not treating the cause — it's treating the symptom.

Functional wellness begins with appreciating the natural ability our body has to heal, just like a plant, and seeking to support that healing process through those foundational principles.

Functional Wellness Practitioners: A Different Look at Lab Tests

At our practice, I often sit down with someone and they tell me that their doctor ran some blood work and the labs came back normal. The person may seem a little upset about that, and I ask them why.

They often say, "Because I don't *feel* normal. I'm still suffering and I still have these symptoms and issues, so why is the doctor telling me that everything is normal when they run my blood work?"

The explanation is actually quite simple: It's because when you get your blood work done here in the United States, your doctor compares all of your values to all of the other people who have had blood work done over the past year — they are looking at the averages placed on a bell-shaped curve, and anything that falls within a specific range is considered normal, and anything that falls outside of that range is considered abnormal.

You should see immediately two problems with this approach to analyzing lab results.

1. Do you want to be compared to the average American citizen?

2. Who do you think is going in to get blood work done?

The answers are, "No, I don't want to be an average American," because most Americans are ill, and, "The people getting blood tests are sick people, and they're on a lot of medications." Those medications artificially change lab values.

So when you go in and get your blood work done, and then your doctor sits you down and says, "Congratulations, everything is normal," what they're really saying is this: "Congratulations, you look like every other sick, medicated person who had their blood work done over the past year."

When functional wellness practitioners like me look at blood testing, we don't simply look at averages — we look at what are called functional lab ranges. These are not based on averages. They are based on what research has shown optimal health looks like. We're actually comparing you to healthy people.

This gives us a much narrower range in which to see where you might fall within normally accepted lab values, and yet fall outside of what is considered optimal. We can get a lot of information about where your health might be starting to shift or deviate, so that we can be proactive and establish preventive methods, rather than wait for a major problem to develop. These functional lab ranges allow us to be proactive and to help you start to make some positive changes immediately.

Recall the story I shared about my grandfather, Herb. I learned two very valuable lessons from him:

1. No matter how much I care about somebody or seek to help them, ultimately it is up to the individual to choose to take action or not.

2. The true solution to our health crisis simply cannot be found in pills.

The second lesson suggests that we need to start thinking differently about our health, and we need to start acting differently. The true solution is actually in education.

In the world of functional wellness, I am able to teach you:

- Why things aren't working

- Exactly what you can be doing from a lifestyle perspective to become proactive

- What you can do to take control of your health

Now that you understand the basics behind why we need to start becoming proactive, the next few chapters discuss some of the most common areas of dysfunction that I encounter with the people I work with.

These chapters cover four specific areas of hormone-related problems that can lead to serious health complications later on in life.

Hormone-related problems tend to affect:

- Sleep
- Digestion
- Energy
- Fat-burning
- Weight loss

The next chapter:

- Explores these specific areas

- Introduces the basics behind each of those hormone systems

- Discusses why they are such a problem

- Explains how we can test for them

- Examines the differences between the conventional approach and the functional wellness approach

CHAPTER
TWO

Adrenal Hormones

THE ADRENAL PERSON

There are four primary hormone groups that can disrupt our overall health and well-being. The first group is your adrenal glands, the hormones that they produce, and the imbalances that can occur when things are not working correctly. It's important to learn about someone dealing with adrenal issues — I refer to them as *the adrenal person* — because this is the health condition that seems to be the most common in our country. I'm going to describe why this has happened, and discuss this particular organ system.

What Do Your Adrenal Glands Do?

Let's first talk about what your adrenal glands do. Your adrenal glands produce three primary types of hormones.

The first hormone is *cortisol*, which is your fight-or-flight hormone. This is the hormone that helps your body adapt to stress. Cortisol is a glucocorticoid, which means that it helps regulate blood sugar levels by stimulating glucose production in the liver and protein breakdown in the muscles. Cortisol is also our get-up-and-go hormone. It helps you wake up in the morning, it helps kick-start your energy for the day, and it helps then regulate your energy and blood sugar levels over the course of the day.

The second type of hormone is *aldosterone*, which is a mineralocorticoid that helps regulate blood pressure through sodium and electrolyte balance.

The third type consists of sex hormones like *testosterone* and *estrogen*. This is especially important for women to understand, because after menopause their ovaries stop producing sex hormones, so the primary source of sex hormones becomes the adrenal glands. If a woman's adrenals were already struggling before menopause, it only gets worse after: she may notice even more symptoms of sex hormones imbalance as the process unfolds, due to the increased demand for sex hormone production that falls on the already stressed adrenal glands. I cover this idea in more detail in the chapter on sex hormones.

How Does the Adrenal Person Look?

I can tell a lot about what type of hormone imbalance might be going on with a particular client as soon as they walk through the front door at the Inspire Wellness Center, because physical appearances can offer a lot of clues about what is going on internally and what hormone system might be falling into a state of dis-ease:

- The adrenal person has a tendency to carry a lot of very stubborn belly fat—the "flop over the belt" type of belly fat. It doesn't matter how many crunches this person does or how much time they spend on the treadmill or exercising, that belly simply will not go away, because the adrenal glands and hormones are actually creating that kind of fat.

- The adrenal person also has a tendency toward skinny legs. If they are exercising and working out, they actually notice that they are burning muscle from their glutes and their thighs and their legs before they lose an ounce of fat from their belly. They end up having skinny, very toned legs and calves, and yet still have protruding belly fat.

- The adrenal person also looks stressed. They look tired, because their adrenal glands are not regulating their energy and their blood sugar very well. This is a person who has the tendency to run around almost as if they're in a constant state of chaos, because their get-up-and-go went up and left, and their fight-or-flight response is in overdrive, creating a lot of stress in their ability to handle daily activities.

How Does the Adrenal Person Feel?

The adrenal person typically feels very stressed because they have lost the ability to adapt to the stressors that daily life presents. They have a tendency to have very low energy, especially first thing in the morning and in the afternoon. The adrenal person may feel that they have a low libido, or a low sex drive. They just don't really have the same get up and go as when they were younger.

The adrenal person craves salty foods. They may also crave sugary foods, but salty food seems to be the most common craving. They're always reaching for that salty snack. The adrenal person also craves caffeine drinks like coffee and soda—they feel that these stimulants make up for what their adrenal glands are no longer doing, to replace some of their need for energy.

The adrenal person feels very tired and yet may have a difficult time falling asleep or staying asleep. A common sign of an adrenal problem is having more energy at night, when it's finally time to go to bed, and not being able to fall asleep. Or having a hard time staying asleep. There can also be a tendency to wake up in the middle of the night. The adrenal person will wake up tired, even after a full night's rest.

If you notice that you have a hard time managing emotional stress compared to other people around you, then this may also be a sign that your adrenals are in crisis. If you notice you're in the same room as someone else and you're both being exposed to the same stressor—maybe it's a boss yelling at you—or you're in 5:00 p.m. traffic and your friend is just cool as a cucumber while you're pulling out your hair, these are signs that your body has lost the ability to adapt to stressors, and that's often a sign of adrenal dysfunction.

Most Americans Have Adrenal Dysfunction

It's important to test and understand how your adrenals function, because most Americans are under stress. We need to properly evaluate adrenal function so that we can start to take proactive measures toward improving our health. Most people with adrenal dysfunction do not have a true disease or pathology related to the adrenal glands. However, the fast-paced American lifestyle does create a state of dis-ease that leads to an accumulation of stress on the adrenal system. That can then lead to a host of other health problems.

With our current lifestyle, most of us live all day, every day, under stress.

Think about how from the moment you wake up:

- You're rushing to get ready for work or school.

- You don't have time to eat breakfast.

- You're caught in slow traffic going to work.

- You're stressed while you're at work.

- You're not able to eat a healthy lunch or even go outside.

- You're unappreciated by your boss and colleagues.

- You drive home in traffic and you're yelling at the other cars on the freeway.

- When you get home:

- You have to make dinner or clean up afterward.

- Your family or friends are stressed out.

- You go to bed crabby and tired after watching a couple of hours of stressful news on TV.

- Finally, you lie wide-awake in bed, worrying about what's coming up the next day.

That is the kind of lifestyle that creates adrenal stress.

Evaluation of Symptoms

Any time I do an educational seminar on belly fat and adrenal stress, I take all of the attendees through a self-evaluation by inviting them to answer a few questions to determine if they have the symptoms that would indicate an adrenal problem.

Go ahead and ask yourself these questions and consider, "Am I an adrenal person?"

1. Do you struggle to manage stress?

2. Do you wake up tired? Do you tell people, "I am not a morning person," or, "Don't talk to me for the first hour of the day?"

3. Do you rely on coffee or caffeinated beverages to get started in the morning, or to keep your energy up throughout the day?

    If you do, that's a sign of adrenal dysfunction, because you are now using that stimulant to replace what your body is no longer producing on its own.

4. Do you crave salty foods?

    As we mentioned earlier, this is a classic sign of adrenal dysfunction.

5. Do you get irritable or agitated between meals, or if you go too long without eating?

    This may be a sign that cortisol is not maintaining your blood sugar levels between meals, and so your blood sugar actually starts to tank, and that can lead to feelings of irritability, or it can create cravings for sugary foods.

6. Do you have an afternoon crash and feel like you're just completely in the pits by the time you reach midafternoon?

7. Do you have more energy at night right before bed, or would you call yourself a night owl?

    If you do, then you may be producing too much cortisol when it's time for you to go to bed, so it's keeping you up at night. There's a neurotransmitter that our body produces, called GABA, and that neurotransmitter helps you fall asleep and stay asleep. Cortisol actually inhibits the release of GABA, which means that if your cortisol is high at night, it will make it more difficult for you to fall asleep and stay asleep.

8. Do you finally fall asleep, but find that you're waking up in the middle of the night?

    If you do, then that means that you may be having spikes of cortisol or that your blood sugar may be getting too low, resulting in the rebound reaction of adrenaline, which can wake you up.

9. Do you have a low sex drive or low libido?

Your adrenal glands produce a lot of your sex hormones, but when you are under too much stress, it will shut off the utilization of those hormones. That's why many people who are under chronic stress find that they have a low libido. Very serious adrenal dysfunction can actually lead to the conversion of sex hormones into other nonuseful hormones, and that can create issues with libido.

HOW DO WE TEST AND CONFIRM THAT THE ADRENAL GLANDS ARE THE PROBLEM?

Saliva Testing for Adrenal Hormones

Traditional testing for adrenal glands typically involves blood tests. Unfortunately, these tests are typically not very helpful, unless you are ruling out actual disease or pathology. The simple reason is that when you do a blood test, you're capturing only one simple view at the very moment when your blood is drawn. However, in the case of adrenal hormones like cortisol, the level should fluctuate a lot over the course of the day. It should be nice and high first thing in the morning when you wake up, and then it should slowly taper off as the day goes on, until it's nice and low at night, so that you can have that release of GABA that helps you fall asleep and sleep through the night. The end result is a healthy circadian rhythm or sleep-wake cycle — and proper sleep patterns.

As you can imagine, if all you do is take one single blood test, all that's going to do is tell you what's going on at that particular moment of the day. It's really not going to give you a complete picture of your overall cortisol pattern.

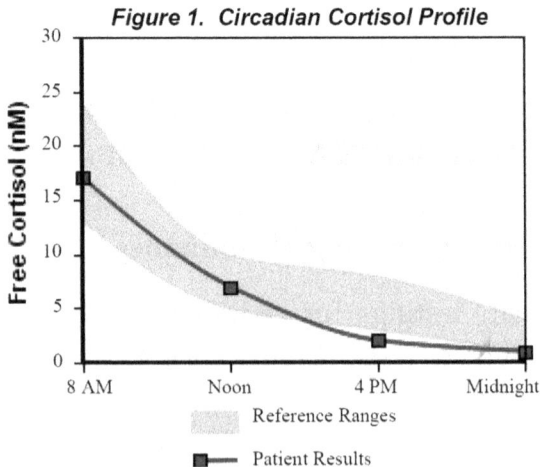

Figure 1. Circadian Cortisol Profile

One of the benefits of saliva testing is that it allows you to take four measurements during one day, which can then be used to track changes in cortisol levels over the course of that day. It's a relatively simple test to perform and it can give us a better indication as to at what time of day the dysfunction might be occurring, and in what way other hormones might be interacting with the adrenal system.

CONVENTIONAL VERSUS FUNCTIONAL AP-PROACHES TO SUPPORTING ADRENAL HEALTH

As I discuss the different hormones and organ systems that are involved with our health and well-being, you're going to find that a common theme keeps reoccurring. The underlying cause of adrenal dysfunction comes down to lifestyle.

I want to remind you of the question I've posed before: If lifestyle is creating disease in your body, at what point do you expect that a chemical or a pill can fix it?

The answer is *never*. So the functional approach to supporting an adrenal problem really does focus around the lifestyle aspect and the stressors that are creating dysfunction in your body.

What Is the Conventional Approach?

Before we go into the functional approach to supporting

adrenal health, let's first briefly cover the conventional medical approach to addressing an adrenal problem. If you have a disease or pathology of the adrenal gland, then you need a medical intervention. If you have a disease like Addison's or Cushing's, there are appropriate medical interventions to manage these conditions. Please don't misunderstand the recommendations that I offer in this book: these are not designed to address true pathologies of the adrenal glands.

However, as I mentioned before, most people with adrenal problems aren't dealing with a true pathology.

They will tell their medical practitioner or physician, "I think I have an adrenal problem because I have these symptoms."

However, if they don't have a disease, then there really isn't much that the medical system can do for that person.

The typical recommendation will be, "Well, you probably just need to relax. Go on a vacation. Take up meditation. Try to eat better, exercise, and do yoga."

All of these ideas may be fine and helpful, but they don't get down to the true underlying problem of why the person is struggling.

Functional Approach: Nutrition

Let's cover a few of the key functional considerations when supporting the adrenal system. When it comes to nutrition, there are two primary issues that need to be addressed.

The first one is digestion. Cortisol is damaging to the digestive lining, so many individuals with adrenal problems will also report digestive problems, such as:

- Acid reflux
- Reactivity to foods
- Gas and bloating after meals (Talbott, 2007)

These individuals will need additional testing to determine the health of their digestive system. If digestion is impaired, an appropriate digestive repair protocol may be required in order to help address that underlying issue and how it's affecting their adrenals. This might include:

- Testing for and eliminating certain foods

- Using supportive supplementation of digestive enzymes, probiotics, or hydrochloric acid when appropriate

- Vitamins, minerals, and herbs to support the body's ability to repair the digestive tract

The second nutrition key is blood sugar. Many individuals with adrenal dysfunction also have blood sugar imbalances. There is more detail about this in the next chapter, but getting on a blood-sugar-healthy diet is absolutely key to helping support the adrenal system and helping the person overcome the cravings that they have for sugary foods, salty foods, and so on.

Functional Approach: Exercise and Lifestyle

Next, let's cover some exercise and lifestyle recommendations. First of all, the adrenal person really needs to sleep for eight hours each night. Even if you have a hard time falling asleep and staying asleep, you need to start setting a schedule that will allow for enough sleep. Try to set a time to go to bed, and then set an alarm to wake up at the same time each morning. This helps support your circadian rhythm, or your sleep-wake cycle. Your circadian rhythm is closely tied in with adrenal function. In order to properly regulate cortisol function throughout the day, you want to make sure that your sleep-wake cycle is in sync.

Also, we need appropriate cortisol release first thing in the morning to start the day off well. We should have about a 50 percent increase in cortisol production within twenty to thirty minutes of awakening in the morning. This is called the Cortisol Awakening Response, which gives us our "get up and go" in the morning.

Symptoms of abnormal Cortisol Awakening Response include:

Difficulty waking up in the morning

Need coffee or nicotine to function in the morning

No appetite in the morning

No motivation in the morning

Lowest energy of the day in the first hour after awakening

Figure 1. Circadian Cortisol Profile

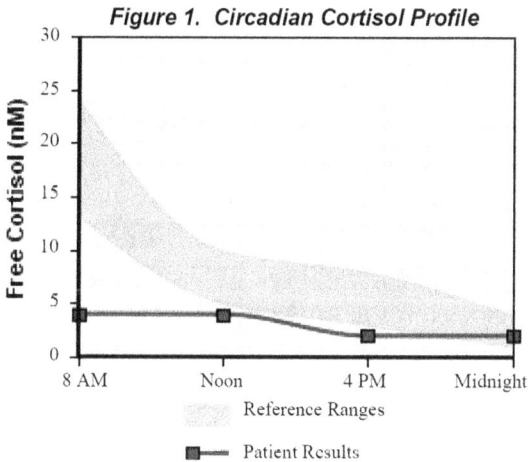

If these symptoms and saliva testing indicate that you have low adrenal function, then first thing in the morning you'll want to engage for five to seven minutes in high-intensity exercise, which will help stimulate cortisol production. It is absolutely critical that these exercises be done first thing in the morning, immediately upon waking, to give you the benefit of the cortisol awakening response.

High-intensity exercise doesn't need to be difficult. For example:

- Grab a jump rope and do 60 seconds of fast jumps, followed by 60 seconds of walking or stretching. Repeat a few times, and you're done.

- Do as many pushups as you can, rest for 60 seconds, then repeat a few times, and you're set for the day.

- Squats, lunges, crunches, dips, or jumping jacks also work to stimulate cortisol.

I do need to add a note of warning to this morning exercise: Do not begin a high-intensity regimen without having proper testing and evaluation done beforehand. If you are an adrenal person, but you are actually in a state of adrenal hyperfunction—meaning that you're producing higher-than-normal levels of cortisol—high-intensity exercise can actually cause overtraining syndrome. This will ultimately make you feel worse, weaker, and even more tired.

One more recommendation for your lifestyle choices: Get off caffeine. It is an adrenal stressor. Caffeine stimulates cortisol production, which may be good in the short term, but over the long term it can be devastating to adrenal health. If you rely on caffeine to get up in the morning, or you rely on caffeine to make it through the day, the best thing that you can do to support your adrenal health is to start to wean yourself off caffeine. I promise you, your body will thank you for it in the long run (Lovallo, 2005).

An "Inspire Wellness" Experience

I feel so much energy right now, I cannot believe it! I was so afraid of where my life was going. I would come home from work and take a nap for one or two hours. I come home now and don't take a nap. I sleep through the night. I hadn't slept through the night in probably ten years! I have no problem getting up in the morning, because I'm not tired; I don't have to drink coffee to get going. My children have told me, "Mom, you have changed so much, you have such a high level of energy, it's like ten years or twenty years ago . . . we have to run to keep up with you."

When you go through this program, you're gonna love it, because the support group is so wonderful. I can't describe how great I feel. My sister talks to me on the phone from Arizona and says, "My gosh, you just sound like a different person."

I am a different person. I have a new life. My life is healthy.

~ Margo C.
Killen, Texas

For most people, adrenal dysfunction ultimately comes down to a combination of lifestyle habits. By appropriately addressing other areas of dysfunction in your body, and then making some simple lifestyle modifications, you can actually do wonders to support your adrenal health.

It's critical that you make these changes and support this organ, because it regulates so many functions in your body, including:

- Producing many of your sex hormones

- Producing aldosterone, which regulates blood pressure

- Producing cortisol, which helps you manage stress and adapt to stress and regulate blood sugar levels

- Communicating with your brain to regulate your sleep-wake cycle and the release of hormones that control thyroid function

It's critical that we take care of our adrenal glands, because unfortunately, adrenal dysfunction sends many people to their graves prematurely.

It causes people to be fat, sick, and run down, and this leads to:

- Blood sugar problems, such as diabetes

- Sex hormone problems, such as low sex drive

- High blood pressure—which can lead to heart disease, heart attacks, or stroke

Adrenal problems cause you to be tired and depressed, because your sleep cycle is out of whack.

An adrenal system that is under stress can wreak havoc on your quality of life.

CHAPTER THREE

Insulin and Blood Sugar

THE INSULIN PERSON

This chapter deals primarily with insulin resistance, which leads to type 2 diabetes. Type 1 diabetes is an autoimmune condition, in which the pancreas can't produce insulin, and is either genetic or acquired very early in life. By contrast, type 2 diabetes is a disease caused by lifestyle and occurs later in life.

We need to talk about insulin because our body's ability to properly utilize insulin or not has actually created a modern-day plague in America: type 2 diabetes. More than one in ten Americans over the age of twenty are diabetic, and over the age of sixty-five that number jumps to more than one in four (Healthline, 2014).

I want to help you understand why this happens and what you can do to protect yourself. I refer to someone dealing with insulin-related issues as *the insulin person*.

What Does Insulin Do?

Almost everything that we eat turns into some form of sugar. Our cells have a natural ability to take up that sugar and use it to create energy. However, if there is a lot of sugar floating around in our blood, and our body wants to get it into our cells faster, it causes our pancreas to release insulin.

Insulin has two primary roles:

1. It turns off the formation of new sugar in the liver.

2. It plugs into receptors on our cells to make it easier for sugar to get into them to be used for energy.

Over time, if there are too many surges of sugar and the resulting insulin spikes, eventually our cells will become resistant to insulin, and blood sugar levels will start to creep up. This is what sets the stage for type 2 diabetes.

What Does the Insulin Person Look Like?

Understanding what the insulin person looks like can actually be a little bit tricky, because while most individuals with insulin resistance will struggle with weight—and this will occur, typically, around the midsection—many diabetics will actually be thin, and will be shocked when they are diagnosed. This was the case with my grandfather, Herb. You heard his story in an earlier chapter.

When I met one of our practice members, Glenn, he had just been diagnosed with type 2 diabetes and prescribed metformin. Glenn was not very overweight and was completely in shock when he was told that he had diabetes. He felt fine, but when the news came, it was a major wake-up call for him. Sadly, one third of all diabetics actually don't even know that they are diabetic, because they may not see or feel any symptoms that would lead them to seek help.

How Does the Insulin Person Feel?

Someone who is developing insulin resistance, or difficulty metabolizing sugar, will often notice the very first thing that happens: more and more craving for sweets. If you're a person who just has to have dessert after meals, that's an indication that sugar is not being metabolized very well in your body. The second thing that the insulin-resistant person will notice is fatigue. They will have a tendency to feel tired throughout the day, but they will especially feel tired after meals. If after you eat, rather than feeling more energetic and as if you can go about and get through your day, you actually feel tired, as if you want to take a nap, then that is a possible indication of an insulin problem as well.

HOW DO WE TEST AND CONFIRM THAT INSULIN IS THE PROBLEM?

If you are concerned that you might have a blood sugar problem or insulin resistance, it is absolutely critical that you get yourself tested to find out. As I mentioned before, this is a modern-day epidemic in our country. This is a topic that is very near and dear to me personally, because not only does my grandfather suffer from diabetes, but my father also has diabetes. And, when I finished my doctorate program in 2011, I was on the road toward an early diagnosis of type 2 diabetes. It became absolutely critical that I start to figure out what wasn't working within my own body, and what it was that had led me down that path, so that I could make appropriate changes.

Fortunately, I was able to do that, even though as a young father at the age of thirty, I was overweight, sick, tired, and stressed. I was able to figure out what wasn't working and turn my lifestyle around in such a fashion that I could improve my health. I now know that I won't ever become diabetic, because I know the kind of lifestyle I need to follow. It all begins with proper testing.

Insulin Resistance Is an Epidemic

We owe it to our kids to teach them how to avoid falling prey to this disease. It is predicted that of all the children born after the year 2000, up to half will become diabetic in their lifetime, because of the American lifestyle (WebMD, 2003).

Complications of diabetes include:

- Weight gain
- Peripheral vascular disease, such as blood vessel destruction
- Neuropathy, or nerve death

Diabetes can lead to:

- Ulcers
- Wounds that won't heal
- Loss of limbs from amputation
- Heart attack
- Stroke
- Alzheimer's disease or dementia

The most common cause of death in diabetics is actually cardiovascular events. Furthermore, diabetes is the number-one cause of developing blindness in adults. Finally, diabetes shortens life expectancy by about ten years.

Evaluation of Symptoms

When it comes to evaluating the symptoms of diabetes or insulin resistance, I want you first to consider the list of complications given previously. If you experience any of the things already discussed, that means there is a good chance that you may be pretty far down the path of insulin resistance. Initially, someone with an insulin or blood sugar problem may not notice any obvious symptoms whatsoever. However, upon closer examination, some of the signs will be there.

Answer these questions for your self-evaluation:

- First, do you crave sweets?

  If you do, then your body has a more difficult time metabolizing sugar.

- Do you feel fatigued after meals?

  If you do, then there's a good chance that your body is having a hard time processing the carbohydrates and the sugars from your meal, so all of your energy is going toward the digestive process.

- Do you feel a need to finish a meal with a dessert or a sweet?

- Do you feel irritable or lightheaded if meals are missed?

  If so, that means your blood sugar may be fluctuating between highs and lows when you eat and between meals.

- Do you have increased thirst or appetite?

- Last, do you experience frequent urination, or make frequent trips to the bathroom?

Blood Test for Insulin Resistance and Diabetes

Traditional blood tests for insulin resistance will look at a fasting blood glucose marker. If the test comes back above 100, that is usually the first indication there may be a blood sugar problem. But that marker is actually not very useful, because it changes every day, and many individuals with an impending blood sugar problem will continue to show regular fasting blood glucose levels, even while they are developing insulin resistance.

Unfortunately, in most medical practices, when someone goes in for a wellness check, the fasting blood glucose is the only marker that is looked at to evaluate a blood sugar problem. Blood sugar problems are often overlooked until they have progressed to a much more serious state.

The condition of having a regular fasting blood glucose level, despite actually having a blood sugar problem, is especially common for individuals with a problem called *functional reactive hypoglycemia*. This person does not tolerate sugar very well. Their blood sugar spikes after eating, but their body quickly overcompensates, and afterwards drives their blood sugar down too far. This is a person who becomes irritable or lightheaded if they go too long without eating, but when you check their fasting blood glucose levels, everything looks normal. They are a blood sugar ticking time bomb.

Hemoglobin A1c — or HbA1c — is a more predictive marker of blood sugar health. It tells us what your average blood sugar levels have been over the past ninety days. Anything above 6.4 is considered diabetic, and anything between 5.7 and 6.4 is prediabetic. This marker can catch blood sugar problems well before fasting blood glucose numbers change.

I recommend that anyone who notices the signs and symptoms of a blood sugar issue ask their healthcare practitioner to check their HbA1c to determine if they are insulin resistant.

CONVENTIONAL VERSUS FUNCTIONAL AP-PROACHES TO SUPPORTING BLOOD SUGAR HEALTH

At the heart of it, diabetes is a disease of lifestyle. The only effective long-term solution is a change in lifestyle. We're going to discuss that as we go into the functional approach to addressing an insulin resistance or blood sugar problem. But first, let's cover what the conventional medical approach is.

What Is the Conventional Approach?

There is a long list of drugs that are used medically to treat diabetes. Categorically, however, they can fit into two primary camps. There are drugs that will artificially lower blood sugar by turning off the body's production of sugar. The most popular drug in this category is metformin. Then there are drugs that artificially lower blood sugar by increasing the uptake of sugar into your cells. Insulin, and all of its analogs, would fit into this category.

All of these medication approaches will, at least for a time, manage blood sugar levels, lower them, and make labs appear better. They will certainly help slow down the progression of some of the complications of diabetes.

Unfortunately, though, neither of these categories of drugs can actually cure diabetes. In fact, prolonged use of insulin actually increases insulin resistance, and causes more weight gain. Although these drugs may make things look a little better for a time, in reality they are nothing more than a Band-Aid. Meanwhile, the disease rages on, silently wreaking havoc on all major organ systems.

I also want to give you a word of caution about drug interactions. Many diabetics are also prescribed cholesterol-lowering drugs such as statins. In fact, just recently, the recommendation for these drugs was increased to cover tens of millions of Americans — even those in good health — in the name of "prevention." However, in 2012, the FDA reported that these cholesterol-lowering medications, these statins, actually raise blood sugar and can trigger diabetes in an otherwise healthy individual, or worsen diabetes in someone who already has the disease (U.S. FDA, 2014).

Additionally, a recent study also indicates that statins speed up the aging process, creating a shorter life expectancy in those who take them (Express, 2015).

It seems that the very drugs we take to manage one condition often end up creating another. There truly is no medical intervention that can compensate for an unhealthy lifestyle.

An "Inspire Wellness" Experience

In 1995 I was diagnosed with full-blown diabetes. I went many years in denial — eating whatever I wanted, skipping my meds, and not exercising. I went on many yo-yo diets and would lose weight only to gain it — and even more — back.

This past year I went in to see my doctor. My blood sugar was a skyrocketing 500, my HbA1c was a 14.8, and my cholesterol and triglycerides were extremely high. My doctor suggested I go on insulin. He explained to me that my health was in danger and I could possibly have a heart attack, stroke, or go blind, as well as having a kidney disease.

Hearing those words put a real scare into me. I decided I needed help and that is when I saw Dr. Botts's advertisement about diabetes. I decided then that I would go to his seminar and find out more about his program, and what I could do to take control not just of my blood sugar, but of my overall health.

Boy, was I glad I did! It has now been six months into the program and I am feeling great. I have lost twenty-five pounds, and gone from a size 14 to a size 8. I just ran follow-up labs with Dr. Botts and my blood sugar is a 117, my HbA1c is now a 5.8, and my cholesterol and triglycerides are in the normal range. It is rewarding to see my numbers going down. I was once taking 2000 milligrams of metformin a day and a twelve-hour extended release of glipizide. I am now off all meds!

Managing diabetes had not been easy for me in the past. Dr. Botts has given me the tools to be successful and it has changed my life for the better.

~ Sonya S.
Jarrell, Texas

The Functional Approach

The first key to unwinding insulin resistance and getting blood sugar under control is putting together the correct nutrition plan. Most things we eat turn into some form of sugar in the body. We need to understand how to balance our diet appropriately to manage that sugar. For the insulin-resistant individual, it's important to learn how to slow down the conversion of food, to give the body a slow, sustainable source of fuel, and to avoid rapid spikes in blood sugar and the resulting insulin surges that follow.

Lean protein, healthy fats, and vegetables really are the staples of a healthy blood sugar diet. Just as a side note, don't worry about fats. The myth of low-fat diets was busted years ago, and dietary fat does not turn into fat in your body.

But do you want to guess what *does* turn into fat?

Carbohydrates.

Carbohydrates are really just another word for sugar. And if carbohydrates are not immediately needed for energy, they are converted and stored away in the body, first as glycogen in the liver and muscles for energy reserves, and then as fat. I like to refer to carbohydrates as either fast carbs, if they are quickly metabolized and have a tendency to create blood sugar spikes, or slow carbs, if they break down more slowly and give long-term, sustainable energy.

Examples of fast carbs are:

- Grains: bread, pasta, rice, and corn
- Starches: potatoes, beans, and peas
- Sugars: sweets, desserts, and sodas

These should all be strictly limited. All other vegetables are great sources of slow carbs, and they don't have much of an impact on blood sugar levels.

For the individual who also wants to lose weight, they should strictly limit fructose consumption. This comes from high-glycemic fruits, high-fructose corn syrup, and common table sugar.

Fructose is a sneaky form of sugar:

- Fructose does not affect insulin levels, which might appear to be good news for a diabetic, but it instead bypasses normal sugar metabolism and goes straight to fat storage.

- Fructose doesn't satisfy the body's craving for sugar.

- Continued exposure to fructose can lead to a condition called leptin resistance, which not only promotes fat storage, but also increases our appetite and our cravings for sugar.

As a side note: Stay away from agave syrup. It was once touted as a great sugar alternative because it is very low in sucrose, the form of sugar that affects insulin production. However, agave syrup contains up to 90 percent fructose. That's right, it's an even higher concentration than high-fructose corn syrup, making it sweeter, more addicting, and even more craviing-inducing!

Under absolutely *no* circumstances should you be replacing sugar with artificial sweeteners.

There is a plethora of research that indicates the following:

- Artificial sweeteners not only trigger insulin resistance, but also create more cravings for sugar.

- They can promote fat storage.

- Some of these sweeteners are toxic not only to our brains, but also to our digestive systems, and can create imbalances in our microflora, the bacteria within our digestive lining.

In the research I've done, the only nonsugar sweetener I've found to be safe for the insulin-resistant individual is stevia. It is natural and there is some research that indicates it may offer some protective benefits for healthy blood sugar levels. But you know how research is; it changes every day. By the time this book gets printed, I may be writing a retraction and telling people to stay away from stevia.

Functional Approach: Exercise and Lifestyle

For blood sugar health, any exercise is better than no exercise at all. But there are some methods of exercise that are better than others. High-intensity interval training has been shown to be the most effective form of exercise for improving blood sugar levels (Tjønna et al., 2008).

In fact, compared to light- and moderate-intensity exercise, high-intensity exercise shows improved growth hormone release for fat burning, opioid response for pain relief, increased insulin receptor sensitivity, and improved immune enhancement (Kessler, Sisson, & Short, 2012).

I do need to issue a warning before I begin describing how to perform high-intensity exercise, because this kind of exercise will also increase the risk of overtraining syndrome, which I mention in the chapter on adrenal health. So I always recommend consulting with a trained healthcare professional before starting a high-intensity exercise routine. It's also a good idea to check in periodically to make sure your routine is having the desired effect, and not creating any new problems.

With high-intensity exercise, it really doesn't matter so much *what* you're doing, but how you are performing the exercise. You can look at the attached chart to determine if what you're doing is a low, moderate, or high-intensity exercise.

Let me give you the summary here: If you can carry on a simple conversation while you're working out, it's not high intensity. So hopping on the treadmill and watching TV while you walk, or talking on your phone, or chatting with the person next to you, is not going to get it done. Also, if you don't break into a sweat within a few minutes, then you are not performing a high-intensity exercise. To summarize, you should be sweaty, winded, and even a little bit sore.

Level of Intensity	Maximum Heart Rate MHR = 220 – your age in years	Physical Cues
Light	40–55% of MHR	Does not induce sweating unless it is a hot, humid day. No noticeable change in breathing.
Moderate	55–69% of MHR	Sweating after 10 minutes. Breathing becomes deeper and more frequent. You can carry on a conversation, but not sing.
High	70% or greater of MHR	Will break a sweat after 3–5 minutes. Breathing is deep and rapid. You can talk only in short phrases.

Source: Datis Kharrazian, 2015.

The Centers for Disease Control recognizes that type 2 diabetes is 100 percent preventable and controllable. It requires a proper understanding of why things aren't working properly in your body, and then applying the right nutrition and lifestyle to put your body in the best position to heal. It's been amazing to work with diabetics in our clinic and help them learn how to take care of themselves.

I mentioned earlier in the chapter than when I met Glenn, he was shocked to find out that he had been diagnosed with diabetes. When we first met, his HbA1c was 7.1. Keep in mind that his *true* HbA1c was even higher, because at that time he was taking metformin, which was artificially lowering the lab results.

As we worked together, within a matter of six weeks Glenn improved his blood sugar levels to the point where his physician took him off metformin. He was completely drug-free within six weeks of changing his lifestyle. When we reran his labs at the three-month mark, his HbA1c was down to 5.9. And we knew that this was his *true* HbA1c, because he was off all medications. After six months, he had lost over fifty pounds, and his HbA1c was down to 5.4. That's better than most people who *don't* have diabetes!

I didn't give Glenn any magic pill. I ordered the correct testing and designed an individualized lifestyle program tailored to his needs that he could easily follow. Then I guided him through the process of making the appropriate changes. As a result, his body did what it does best — *heal*.

Truly, the only solution to this diabetes epidemic is in health education and lifestyle changes.

CHAPTER
FOUR

Estrogen and Other Sex Hormones

THE ESTROGEN PERSON

The purpose of this chapter is not to address pathology related to sex hormones such as estrogen, but to discuss the ways in which many people develop imbalances in this delicate system of hormones through the accumulated stresses of our modern-day lifestyle.

What Is Estrogen and How Is It Formed?

There are three types of estrogen that our body produces:

1. **Estrone (E1)** is the primary estrogen after menopause, and it is produced primarily by the adrenal glands and fat cells.

2. **Estradiol (E2)** is the most common form of estrogen, found in menstruating and non-pregnant females.

3. **Estriol (E3)** is the primary form of estrogen during pregnancy.

All three of these forms of estrogen are made from cholesterol, which is formed into androstenedione and then converted into estrogen. Some estrogen goes through a middle step of first forming testosterone, and then being converted to estrogen by an enzyme called aromatase.

What Does the Estrogen Person Look Like?

Ruling out true pathology of an estrogen or sex hormone problem, there are three primary estrogen imbalances that we will see, clinically, day to day:

1. The first one is menstruating women with an estrogen dominance. High levels of estrogen promote fat storage in the chest and thighs, so this individual will have a truly difficult time losing weight around their hips and thighs. It doesn't matter how much time they spend on the stair climber, the treadmill, or whatever. That fat is not going away as long as there is an estrogen dominance.

2. The second form is menopausal women with low estrogen. This woman may look very thin, or follow a very strict diet, which means she doesn't have adequate fat stores to produce the

less potent form of estrogen, estrone. Remember that estrone is the primary estrogen after menopause, and it is produced primarily by adrenal glands and fat cells. Very thin women are more likely to suffer with symptoms of low estrogen while going through menopause, because they don't have the fat stores to create that form of estrogen. Or a menopausal woman may have an adrenal body type with stubborn belly fat. Their adrenal glands have been stressed for a very long time, but they got by before menopause because their ovaries were still producing most of their estrogen. The symptoms of low estrogen have only started to show now that their ovaries are no longer helping out, and all of the hormone production is now falling on the already overstressed adrenal glands.

3. The third primary estrogen imbalance that we find is in men with low testosterone. I mentioned earlier that some of our estrogen is produced by the enzyme aromatase, which is present in testosterone. A very common reason for men to be deficient in testosterone is not due to simple underproduction of testosterone, but rather the active conversion of testosterone into estrogen by this enzyme. And the most common reason for this conversion to be stimulated or upregulated in men is insulin resistance or

diabetes (Grossman et al., 2013). So the man with an estrogen body type looks very similar to the insulin body type, with mid-section weight gain and increased fat around the chest area.

Just a quick note on women with insulin resistance: In women with blood sugar problems, the opposite conversion actually takes place. They will actively convert estrogen into testosterone, and will experience the symptoms of a resulting estrogen deficiency, such as facial hair growth, hair loss on the top of the head, and low libido (Brand et al., 2011). In women, this increases the risk for cancer, especially in organs that require higher levels of estrogen, like ovaries, endometrium, and breasts (Suba, 2012). This correlation is also found in women with polycystic ovarian syndrome, which creates high levels of testosterone, and a higher risk for diabetes (Sheehan, 2004).

How Does the Estrogen Person Feel?

A person with a sex hormone imbalance will likely feel the following symptoms:

- Changes in libido, such as low sex drive
- Changes in energy level and mood
- More depressed or emotional
- Loss of motivation and self-confidence

Menstruating women may also notice:

- Changes in cycle length

- Extreme changes to mood and emotions at different times in cycle

- A sense that most of the month is spent in total chaos, with only a few days of peace between cycles

Menopausal women who are struggling with an estrogen imbalance may experience hot flashes, night sweats, and fluctuations in body temperature.

Because it is very common for men with blood sugar problems to experience symptoms of low testosterone and increased estrogen, they may then notice issues with:

- Low libido
- Erectile dysfunction
- Low motivation and confidence

Men with these low testosterone and increased estrogen issues have a tendency to become "soft and squishy," both on the inside and the outside.

Recently, testosterone hormone replacement therapy has become a very popular "quick fix" for symptoms of low testosterone, or low "T" as it is called in advertisements. However, I want to add a word of caution before you rush out to use this therapy.

Initially, men who use testosterone therapy may feel better, but over time, many of them start slowly developing signs of high estrogen:

- Shrinking gonads
- Low libido
- Increase in breast tissue

The reason for this is that their body's current physiological state is actively converting testosterone into estrogen via the enzyme aromatase. Without addressing the underlying conversion problem, pumping the body full of testosterone is like throwing fuel on the fire. The body will actively convert this influx of testosterone into estrogen, ultimately worsening the problem. If you want a good example of this problem, just look at older body builders who have started to develop feminine features. They likely overutilized testosterone therapy for many years.

HOW DO WE TEST AND CONFIRM THAT ES-TROGEN IS THE PROBLEM?

If you believe that you may have a sex hormone imbalance, it's absolutely critical for you to have proper testing done before engaging in any type of treatment or therapy. The reason this is so important is because the overuse of these hormones, as I mentioned earlier, can actually end up creating more problems.

Understand the High-Risk Groups

You are at a high risk of developing a sex hormone imbalance if:

- You have blood sugar problems like insulin resistance or diabetes

- You suffer from adrenal dysfunction (which we cover in the previous chapter)

- You experience thyroid problems (which we cover in the next chapter)

- You are perimenopausal or menopausal

- You have certain chronic health issues, such as polycystic ovarian syndrome, uterine fibroids, or endometriosis

Evaluation of Symptoms

When evaluating for symptoms, we are going to consider three different groups: menstruating women, menopausal women, and men.

Menstruating women, ask yourselves the following questions:

- Is your cycle length irregular or changing?

- Do you experience pain or cramping during your periods?

- Do you notice changes in blood flow, either too little or too heavy?

- Do you experience breast pain and swelling during menses?

- Do you experience pelvic pain during menses?

- Are you irritable and depressed?

- Do you notice problems with acne?

- Have you noticed increased facial hair growth?

- Have you noticed hair loss and thinning in other areas?

Women who are in menopause can ask these questions:

- Do you still have uterine bleeding?

- Do you experience hot flashes or mental fogginess?

- Have you noticed less interest in sex?

- Have you noticed mood swings or depression?

- Do you experience vaginal dryness or pain during intercourse?

- Do you have increased facial hair growth and acne?

Men, consider these questions:

- Have you noticed a decreased libido or decreased number of morning erections?

- Do you have decreased fullness of erections or difficulty maintaining an erection?

- Do you experience mental fatigue?

- Do you have an inability to concentrate?

- Do you suffer episodes of depression?

- Have you noticed unexplained muscle soreness?

- Do you have unexplained weight gain? Have you noticed increased fat around the chest and hips?

- Do you have sweating attacks?

- Do you feel more emotional than in the past?

These are all symptoms of what we call *andropause* in men.

Saliva Testing for Sex Hormones

I prefer saliva testing for sex hormones for a couple of reasons. First, it allows us to see what hormones are available at the tissue level. For the person who's already on hormone therapy, it allows us to see what might be getting stored away in their tissues from what they're taking. Clients on hormone therapy are often shocked when they sit down to review the results of the saliva hormone testing with me and the results show high levels of the very hormone they were told was deficient.

Hormones have a widespread impact across the whole body. Traditional blood testing may sometimes miss part of the picture. For menstruating females, saliva testing offers an easier way to test sex hormones during an entire month's cycle. Since there is a lot of fluctuation and variation throughout the cycle, this can allow us to get a better picture. It can offer some valuable insights into why a cycle might be longer or shorter than usual, why the person may be experiencing severe PMS, or why they are having difficulty ovulating or conceiving.

CONVENTIONAL VERSUS FUNCTIONAL AP-PROACHES TO SUPPORTING SEX HORMONE HEALTH

In cases of disease or pathology, I always recommend

conventional medical treatment. However, most people who deal with sex hormone imbalances will find, upon further investigation, that the true underlying cause of dysfunction can actually be traced back to other organ systems not working in communication with each other, or other lifestyle factors that they actually have control over. So before we jump in and start talking about what the functional wellness approach would be for some of these issues, let's talk about the conventional treatment that is typically offered for the nonpathological patient.

What Is the Conventional Approach?

For everyone who isn't dealing with pathology, the typical medical approach is to run a blood test, and then prescribe hormones to replace the deficiency. The vehicle for delivery will likely be in the form of an oral medication or some type of topical lotion or cream.

Since we've been focusing primarily on estrogen in this chapter, let's talk a little bit about estrogen medication. Oral estrogens are converted into estrone by the liver. Estrone is considered by some to be a bad form of estrogen and it is hypothesized to be the source of estrogen's cancer-causing properties. Oral estrogens also block growth hormone from activating the liver to produce what's called insulin-like growth factor, or IGF-1. IGF-1 helps increase energy and a sense of well-being. Oral estrogens may offer some benefits for improving parameters related to heart disease, such as raising HDL, which is considered the good form of cholesterol. It may also offer some antioxidants.

Topical forms of estrogen run the risk of being stored away in tissues, especially fat cells, as I mention earlier. Blood tests may show normal levels of estrogen, but a saliva test will show that the estrogen levels are through the roof because the hormone is accumulating in peripheral tissues. Anyone who is on a topical form of estrogen or hormone therapy runs that risk.

You also run the risk of exposing loved ones to these hormones if you take them in topical form. A colleague of mine shared a surprising experience: She was working with a couple and the husband was using a topical testosterone to treat the symptoms of low testosterone, and the wife was using an estrogen cream for low estrogen. When the saliva hormone testing came back, the husband was still low in testosterone but through the roof in estrogen, and conversely the wife was high in testosterone but still low in estrogen. They were exposing each other to their hormone treatment, just by sharing the same bed! Because the underlying conversion pathways were still dysfunctional in their bodies, the treatments were having effects that were the reverse of what was desired.

Another quick note on drug interactions: I can't say enough about the problems that cholesterol-lowering medications have created in our society. Consider this: Hormones are made from cholesterol.

If you take a drug that lowers cholesterol, what impact do you think that will have on your body's natural ability to produce these hormones?

It should come as no surprise to you, then, that research has linked cholesterol medication use with the development of low libido, erectile dysfunction, and other forms of sexual dysfunction.

An "Inspire Wellness" Experience

As Maria approached the age of forty, her dream of becoming a mother seemed to be fading. She had already faced many health challenges — leukemia, diabetes, polycystic ovarian syndrome, and autoimmune thyroid disease. Her doctors had told her that she would never have kids. We started working together, supporting her health through nutrition and lifestyle. Six weeks later, she was pregnant, completely naturally! Throughout Maria's pregnancy, her doctor was amazed at how healthy her blood work and hormone levels looked. Nine months later, Maria gave birth to a beautiful, healthy girl. A little over a year later, she gave birth again, this time to a healthy boy. I am continually amazed by the incredible ability our bodies have to heal, if they are provided with the right support.

Functional Support for Sex Hormones

From a lifestyle perspective, the first and most important thing to do when dealing with sexual hormone disruption is to stay away from the chemicals and the environmental toxins that disrupt the formation and metabolizing of these hormones. These are what we call endocrine disruptors. We live in a chemical-laden wasteland, and unfortunately, we can't eliminate all exposure, but we should still do everything we can to clean up our immediate environment as much as possible.

- **BPA**: This endocrine disrupter, which is found in plastic and in the linings of cans, mimics estrogen in the body and has been found to induce insulin resistance (Alonso-Magdalena et al., 2006). Get plastic out of your house. Use glass instead, and if you must use plastic, don't heat it up, because this will leach chemicals into the food or liquid that you are storing.

- **Atrazine**: Found in herbicides, this substance has been linked to breast tumors, delayed puberty, prostate inflammation in animals, and prostate cancer in people. Researchers have even discovered that exposure to low levels of atrazine can turn male fish, amphibians, and reptiles into females that produce completely viable eggs (Hayes et al., 2011). Get rid of these herbicides.

- **Phthalate**: Found in plastic and listed as "fragrance" in personal care products and many other household products, phthalate can trigger cell death in testicular cells. Studies have linked phthalate to hormone changes, lower sperm count, less mobile sperm, birth defects in the male reproductive system, obesity, diabetes, and thyroid irregularities. Any item that lists "fragrance" as an ingredient is just disguising the role of phthalate in its contents (Pflieger-Bruss, Schuppe, & Schill, 2004).

- **Organophosphate pesticides**: Neurotoxic organophosphate compounds that were produced by the Nazis for chemical warfare during World War II were fortunately never used. However, after the war, American scientists used the same chemistry to develop pesticides that target the nervous system of insects. Multiple studies have linked these chemicals to problems with brain development, behavior, fertility, low testosterone (Jaga & Dharmani, 2003), and altering thyroid hormone levels (Lacasaña et al., 2010).

- **Glycol ethers**: Found in paints, cleaning products, brake fluid, and cosmetics, glycol ethers can damage fertility and unborn children. Exposure is also linked to low sperm count (Cherry et al., 2008) and increased asthma and allergies (Choi et al., 2010).

- **Skin care products**: Most makeup products and lotions are hidden sources of sex hormones, among other toxic chemicals, especially if they advertise any type of anti-aging, gravity-defying, or skin-toning benefits. Companies are not required to list these ingredients as long as they fall below the threshold for required listing. The words "proprietary blend" can hide a lot of nasty ingredients. In fact, these estrogenic chemicals have been detected in breast tumors, suggesting their potential role in the development of breast cancer (Harvey & Darbre, 2004).

We teach a class at our clinic called "Healthy Home," in which we give our clients access to resources and strategies for cleaning up their houses and limiting exposure to chemicals. A great place to start on your own is the Environmental Working Group (www. ewg.org). If you are curious about the ingredients in any of your household cleaning products or skin care products, their website can offer information and offer alternatives and methods of eliminating as many of them from your life as possible.

Here are a few ideas to help you reduce your exposure to these harmful endocrine disruptors:

- **Buy organic**. Organic produce and beef reduce your exposure to added hormones, pesticides, and fertilizers. In addition to having harmful chemicals, traditional meats are also loaded with antibiotics. In fact, research has shown that upwards of 50 percent of nonorganic meats at the grocery store have measurable levels of antibiotics in them, which then end up in us once we eat them.

- **Buy fresh**. Packaged and processed foods are common sources of chemicals that are endocrine disruptors.

- **Filter your water**. Our tap water is contaminated with chemicals and prescription medications. These things are *not* removed at the treatment facility. Unfortunately, buying bottled water may not be any better. For one, the water has been sitting in a plastic bottle in the back of a hot delivery truck, so chemicals are likely to have leached out of the plastic. Second, much of the bottled water comes from a common source like tap water, anyway.

- **Use a vacuum cleaner with a HEPA filter**. Our furniture and carpets have a lot of chemicals and fire retardants in them. We may not be able to change that, but we can at least remove as much of the contaminated dust as possible from our homes through regular cleaning.

- **Use natural cleaning products.** If it gets on your hands or on the surfaces where you prepare and eat meals, then it will end up in your body. Use all-natural alternatives available at health food stores to limit this.

- **Use natural skin care products.** The Environmental Working Group (www.ewg. org/research/dirty-dozen-list-endocrine-disruptors) and other websites and natural foods stores can help you to find what you need.

I know this may all seem overwhelming at first glance, but hopefully it's also startling you awake to the fact that you are being exposed to a high level of toxic chemicals on a daily basis, many of which have been proven to disrupt hormone production in our bodies. So it should come as no surprise that so many people suffer with subclinical sex hormone dysfunction, and many children go through early puberty, delayed puberty, and all kinds of different hormone problems related to our exposure to endocrine disruptors.

One last note: There are also all-natural herbs and supplements that can be used to support the body's ability to produce and metabolize sex hormones. Ultimately, these products are just concentrated foods, but they can have an incredible impact on the body's function. However, no amount of supplements can make up for an unhealthy lifestyle or a toxic environment. Also, I'm purposely not giving you any specific recommendations for herbs and supplements, because I always recommend proper testing and the guidance of a healthcare professional who is trained in a functional wellness approach before utilizing any supplement support. Don't self-diagnose and don't self-medicate.

Treating the Body as a Whole

I am always very wary of people who rush into hormone replacement therapy thinking that it will solve all their problems.

Many people imagine, "If my lab tests show an estrogen deficiency, then I should just take estrogen. If a little bit makes me feel better, then a lot will make me feel great!"

Hormones have a widespread effect throughout the entire body, and they exist in a very delicate balance. Supplementing hormones will almost always have a butterfly effect on other systems of the body.

Hormone replacement may be appropriate but, if used, I always recommend addressing the underlying dysfunction, and having an "escape strategy" for eventually weaning off of the hormone therapy. Once you have ruled out pathology through conventional medical testing, many sex hormone imbalances are due to other organ systems not working well together.

Let's review some of the key points of how the whole body needs to work together for proper sex hormone function.

First, blood sugar problems like insulin resistance and diabetes can change the conversion process of sex hormones so that men will have a tendency to convert testosterone into estrogen, and women will convert estrogen into testosterone. Getting blood sugar under control is critical. You can review the chapter on insulin for more information on how to address that issue.

Second, the brain controls everything, and everything else that goes on in the body affects the brain. Your hypothalamus and your pituitary gland in your brain control the release of hormones, which then regulate hormones in the rest of the body. Additionally, everything else that's going on in your body has a feedback mechanism to the brain. Remember this point, because we will talk about it again, in the next chapter on the thyroid gland. If the body and brain are not communicating, hormone release will not happen. This connection is called the hypothalamic-pituitary-gonadal axis.

Third, adrenal glands help produce sex hormones, and most of us have stressed out our adrenal glands.

Remember, this is a common cause of sex hormone problems in women after menopause, because their adrenal glands are now the primary source of estrogen. Also, chronic exposure to cortisol—the primary stress hormone in the adrenal glands—inhibits hormone release in the brain. An adrenal repair program is often appropriate for someone with a sex hormone imbalance. You can refer to the chapter on the adrenals and cortisol for more information.

Finally, the liver makes cholesterol, which is then used to make hormones. The liver plays a key role in converting and metabolizing most of our hormones. Also, our liver detoxifies the body, and eliminates from our system the toxins and chemicals that we are exposed to. Over time, most of us end up with a liver that is overworked. That is why it is a good idea to periodically detoxify your liver. All of the clients who work with us at the Inspire Wellness Center start their program by following a doctor-led detox protocol, to support proper liver detoxification.

The topic of sex hormones is such a huge topic that I could never do it justice in just one chapter. But I hope that this has given you an overview into how many of the lifestyle stressors and substances that we are exposed to can disrupt our ability to utilize these hormones. Truly, volumes have been written—and could still be written—on this topic.

The purpose of this chapter is by no means meant as a diagnostic tool or as a specific treatment plan to address these issues, but rather as a starting point to understand why it's so important for you to start looking into these issues, and to start taking care of yourself.

CHAPTER FIVE

Thyroid Hormones

THE THYROID PERSON

Thyroid dysfunction and thyroid symptoms are very common, especially in the United States and among women. Men also struggle with thyroid symptoms, but you'll notice in this discussion that it is primarily an issue that women face today. In fact, studies suggest that up to 10 percent of women over the age of sixty have some form of hypothyroidism (Nygaard, 2016).

In this chapter, I will be focusing on hypothyroidism, or low thyroid function, because that is the most common form of thyroid dysfunction that we see. Hypothyroidism is also more successfully managed through functional wellness and lifestyle support as opposed to hyperthyroidism, or high thyroid function, which often does require medical intervention. Let's jump in and talk about what thyroid hormones do.

What Do Thyroid Hormones Do?

Thyroid hormones plug into the DNA of every cell in the body to affect protein synthesis. You can't say that about any other hormone (Nussey & Whitehead, 2001). Thyroid hormones also support every major function of the body, which means that if thyroid hormones are balanced, everything else seems to work pretty well. But if thyroid hormones are not working, then everything slows down. One of my colleagues compares the thyroid to the gas pedal on your car: If it is working, then the entire engine runs smoothly, everything moves, and the car gets down the road. If the thyroid is not working, it's like taking your foot off the gas pedal: everything slows down.

Different systems are supported by the thyroid, including:

- **Bone metabolism:** Patients with low thyroid function who use hormone replacement therapy are at higher risk of bone loss leading to osteoporosis (Garlin et al., 2014).

- **The immune system:** Thyroid hormones help regulate the immune system.

- **Brain and nervous system:** "Brain fog" is a commonly reported symptom from thyroid patients, in which they can't seem to think clearly. They report feeling like they are in a haze or a fog.

- **Gastrointestinal function:** Remember, when the thyroid isn't working, *everything* slows down, including digestion.

- **Liver and gallbladder function:** Low thyroid function can slow down liver metabolism pathways. Also, there is an established relationship between thyroid function and the development of gallstone disease (Völzke, Robinson, & John, 2005).

- **Growth and sex hormones:** Problems with low libido and imbalances in estrogen and testosterone are very common with thyroid issues. Problems with growth hormones can also affect your metabolism and your ability to burn fat. Metabolism comes to a screeching halt, and no matter how much the person works out, they just can't seem to lose the weight.

- **Insulin and glucose metabolism:** Low thyroid function can cause metabolic syndrome, which opens the door to insulin resistance and diabetes (Garduño-Garcia et al., 2010). Metabolic syndrome also puts the individual at higher risk for developing obesity (Ambrosi et al., 2010). Tying it all together: Low thyroid function slows down your ability to get sugar from your blood stream into your cells. This can create symptoms of hypoglycemia (lightheaded, irritable) even though blood sugar levels may be normal. To compensate, the adrenals release cortisol (the adrenal hormone) to raise blood sugar levels. High cortisol then further suppresses thyroid function, and the cycle repeats. So a chronic thyroid problem can easily turn into a blood sugar and adrenal problem as well (Kalra, Gopalakrishnan, Unnikrishnan, & Sahay, 2014).

- **Healthy cholesterol levels:** Hypothyroidism affects LDL cholesterol receptors in the liver, which can cause increased cholesterol levels in the blood (Shin & Osborne, 2003).

- **Proper stomach acid:** Many low thyroid patients also suffer from acid reflux. The cause of this is likely quite different from what you might think. I want to cover this one in just a little bit more detail, because many people do suffer unnecessarily with acid reflux, and they end up on medication for life, or Tums, antacids, and so on.

If you have acid reflux, you've probably been told that you are producing *too much* stomach acid, which is causing your reflux symptoms. If you are a hypothyroid patient, you are actually likely producing *too little* stomach acid, resulting in reflux type symptoms. Let me explain what I mean by this. Remember that with low thyroid function, everything in the body slows down. That includes digestive function, so your bowels move slower, and your stomach actually produces less acid to help digestion (Elbert, 2010). That's right, you will actually form *less* stomach acid when thyroid function is low. When you eat a piece of chicken, for example, it will sit in your stomach like a brick and won't be properly broken down because of low stomach acid and low gut motility. Then, bacteria that should have been killed by your stomach acid will start to feed off the chicken, and they will release toxins and acid as they feed. These noxious chemicals splash up into your esophagus, and you experience reflux.

If you take a proton pump inhibitor like Nexium, Prevacid, or any number of these medications that shut off your body's ability to produce stomach acid, it will probably make you feel better in the short term, but what do you think it will do for the problem in the long term?

Fix it?

Nope. It will actually make the problem worse. In many cases of acid reflux related to low thyroid function, successful management actually requires *increasing* stomach acid in order to support proper breakdown of food and destruction of invading bacteria.

What Does the Thyroid Person Look Like?

In terms of physical appearance, low thyroid patients typically struggle with weight gain; not all, but most. They will have a tendency to carry weight everywhere across the body. Remember, everything slows down with low thyroid function, and this includes metabolism and muscle development.

I know I'm talking to a thyroid patient when they tell me that they are eating nothing but salads and gaining weight.

Or they might say, "I went on a fad diet with my friend. She lost fifteen pounds, I lost fifteen ounces."

The thyroid patient may work out for an hour, six days a week, just to maintain their weight, and if they take even one day off, they will start to gain weight again. If this sounds like you, I want to reassure you that it is not your fault. It doesn't matter how much you count the calories, or how much you work out, this thyroid hormone balance is effectively derailing all of your best efforts at losing weight, burning fat, or building muscle.

A thyroid person will often notice hair loss or thinning

on the top of their head. Thinning of the outer third of the eyebrows is another classic sign of hypothyroidism. If you look in the mirror, and your eyebrows look absolutely beautiful and you haven't had to pluck them in months, that might actually not be a good sign.

How Does the Thyroid Person Feel?

Low thyroid patients usually feel tired and sluggish. They might require excessive amounts of sleep just to function. Another common symptom of hypothyroidism is low bowel function, like I mentioned earlier. This person may go days without a bowel movement, but then they may also experience alternating bouts of constipation and diarrhea, or gas and bloating after meals, especially if they have an undiagnosed immune reaction to certain foods in their diet, or if they have an imbalance of the bacteria in their gut.

Headaches are another common symptom of low thyroid function, especially headaches in the morning that then wear off as the day goes on. Many low thyroid patients experience episodes of depression, mood swings, lack of motivation, or anxiety and nervousness.

Another common symptom is cold hands and feet—a low thyroid person has a tendency to be cold all the time. I know I'm getting ready to do a thyroid consult if it's the middle of July, I walk out into the waiting room, and I see that the next patient is wearing a sweatshirt. This person may sometimes feel their hands and feet are cold (or they feel cold all over), and then at other times experience night sweats or hot flashes. Their body temperature has wild fluctuations. This could also be a symptom of menopause, depending on age, but many thyroid patients also experience this.

Finally, the thyroid person experiences insomnia.

Now, isn't that a sick joke?

You wake up tired, you struggle to make it through the day, you're exhausted when you get home, and then when it's finally time to go to bed, you can't sleep. As you can see, for the person struggling with thyroid symptoms, this can be a real challenge. It can affect all of your daily activities and your quality of life and ability to get out and do the things that you want to.

When I first met Tammye, she sat down and, in tears, told me that she was just struggling to get by as a wife and a mother. She could hardly make it through the day at work. When it was time to come home, she had no energy to make meals for her family. She loved cooking, but she just couldn't do it, so she'd been getting drive-through meals for her family. Then, when the weekend came, she would literally sleep all day on Sunday, just so that she could then make it through the next week.

As you can imagine, this created a lot of stress for her, and obviously upset her family a great deal.

Once we started to finally address some of the underlying causes behind why she was suffering, it was amazing to see the incredible turnaround that occurred within a matter of just a couple of months. Tammye was able to get back to doing the things that she enjoyed doing, cooking and preparing meals for her family.

For her, the true eye-opener was when her daughter said, "Mom, it's so good to have you back. I'm so happy to be able to go out and be doing things with you again on Sunday, because you don't have to sleep all day anymore."

With a list of symptoms like this, it should come as no surprise that many thyroid patients are at their wits' end trying to find a solution for this problem.

HOW DO WE TEST AND CONFIRM THAT THE THYROID GLAND IS THE PROBLEM?

In order to understand if you truly have a thyroid problem, you want to first evaluate the way you look and feel. If you have a lot of symptoms, then there's a pretty high likelihood that you do have a thyroid condition, regardless of what your lab tests might show. First, in order to understand how to properly evaluate the thyroid, we need to talk a little bit about how thyroid hormone physiology works. Let's jump in and cover that.

Understanding Thyroid Hormone Physiology

Many individuals who sit down with me are very frustrated.

They tell me, "My doctor ran the blood tests, he put me on thyroid hormones, and then he ran a follow-up test and told me that everything was fixed. Yet, I still have thyroid symptoms. What's going on?"

What I tell that person is, "Well, you need to understand a little bit about how thyroid hormones are actually produced and used, because many people *will* continue to suffer with thyroid symptoms even if they are taking a thyroid hormone medication."

So let's talk a little bit about the physiology of how thyroid hormones are produced, and I think you'll start to understand why many people still have thyroid symptoms.

Your hypothalamus, which is in your brain, sends a hormone called *thyrotropin-releasing hormone*, or TRH, to the pituitary gland, which is also in your brain.

The pituitary gland then releases *thyroid-stimulating hormone*, or TSH, to activate the thyroid gland. TSH stimulates thyroid peroxidase, or TPO, to create thyroid hormones. The thyroid gland then produces two forms of hormones: T3 and T4. T3 is the active, usable form of thyroid hormone, so if your body were a car, T3 would be the gasoline that makes it run. T3 accounts for only about 7 percent of the hormones produced by the thyroid. T4 is the inactive, unusable form of thyroid hormone. This would be like crude oil. Even though your car can't run on it, the crude oil can be refined or converted into gasoline, and then it can be used. T4 makes up about 93 percent of the hormones produced by the thyroid gland.

You might be asking yourself, "Why would my thyroid make mostly the crude oil, or inactive form, of the thyroid hormone?"

The reason is that thyroid hormones are very powerful, and too much can be life-threatening. In order to protect yourself, your thyroid makes mostly the inactive form, T4 (or crude oil), and then your body converts it into the active T3 (or gasoline) as your body feels the need for it. Let's talk briefly about how this conversion from T4 to T3 takes place.

Ultimately, only about 60 percent of T4 will be converted into T3, and most of this conversion takes place in the liver. Obviously, you need a properly functioning liver in order to convert thyroid hormones. Another 20 percent can be converted to active T3 in the digestive tract, in the presence of healthy bacteria and proper digestive function. If the brain is signaling proper thyroid stimulation, the thyroid is making enough hormones, and the liver and gut are able to convert those hormones, then proper thyroid function can be achieved. As you can see, though, there is a lot more going on than just whether or not the thyroid is actually making enough hormones.

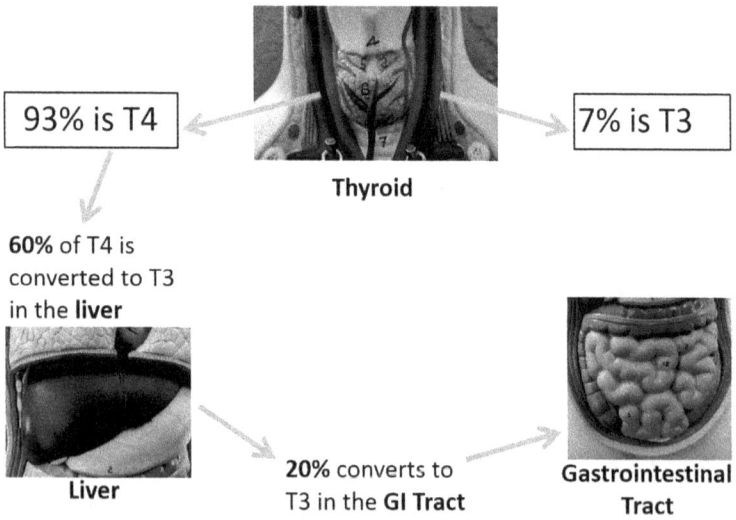

93% is T4

7% is T3

Thyroid

60% of T4 is converted to T3 in the **liver**

Liver

20% converts to T3 in the **GI Tract**

Gastrointestinal Tract

Ninety Percent of Thyroid Problems Are Not Thyroid Problems

The reason I say that 90 percent of thyroid problems are not actually thyroid problems is because blaming an underactive thyroid gland for symptoms is an overly simplistic explanation. In fact, most forms of hypothyroidism involve other organ systems, which are the underlying causes of thyroid dysfunction. Let's take a look at some of the most common causes of thyroid symptoms:

- Primary hypothyroidism
- Hypothyroidism due to low pituitary function
- Thyroid underconversion
- Thyroid-binding globulin elevation
- Thyroid resistance
- Autoimmune thyroid disease, or Hashimoto's disease

The first one is *primary hypothyroidism*. This is the classic form of low thyroid function, which actually can be blamed on a sluggish thyroid gland. Lab tests will show a high TSH with low thyroid hormone production. This form accounts for about 10 percent of thyroid cases, and is also the only form of hypothyroidism that is successfully managed with traditional hormone replacement therapy.

The second one that we want to talk about is *hypothyroidism due to low pituitary function*.

Do you remember where TSH comes from?

That's right, the pituitary gland.

Consider this for a moment: What if your pituitary gland weren't functioning at its optimum?

This could result in decreased release of TSH, which would cause decreased stimulation of the thyroid gland, which would lead to decreased production of thyroid hormone. In this case, the real problem is your pituitary gland not stimulating enough thyroid production. The most common reason for decreased release of TSH from the pituitary is adrenal dysfunction, which creates a negative feedback loop that inhibits pituitary function. In this case, the thyroid problem is actually an adrenal problem; more specifically, a hypothalamic-pituitary-adrenal axis problem. (Try saying that five times fast!)

The third condition is *thyroid underconversion*. This is a dysfunction in the conversion pathway of T4 to T3 that I covered earlier. Even if you have healthy levels of inactive T4, if the liver or digestive system is not functioning properly you may not be converting T4 into the active form, T3. People often ask me why their thyroid medication doesn't seem to be fixing their symptoms. In many cases, the answer is, at least in part, thyroid underconversion.

Here's why: The most commonly prescribed thyroid medications—synthroid or levothyroxine—are synthetic forms of T4, the inactive thyroid hormone. These synthetic hormones can be converted into T3 and utilized by the body, but in many cases, this does not happen. It's like pumping yourself full of crude oil hoping that the car will run, when the ability to refine it into gasoline is impaired. In this case, the thyroid problem is in fact a liver and digestive problem.

The next possibility is *thyroid-binding globulin elevation*. Thyroid-binding globulins do exactly what their name describes: They bind up thyroid hormones, then carry them to where they need to go and release them to the appropriate tissue. However, if you have too many of these binding globulins, then as soon as one releases the thyroid hormone, another one comes and picks it up, so the hormones never arrive where they need to go. Elevated binding globulins are most often the result of high levels of estrogen in the body (Santin & Furlanetto, 2011). This can come from contraceptive use, estrogen hormone therapy, skin care products, or any of the other estrogen problems listed in the previous chapter. In this case, the thyroid problem is actually an estrogen problem.

Next is *thyroid resistance*. In the same way that the cells in a diabetic become resistant to insulin, the cells in a hypothyroid patient may eventually develop a resistance to thyroid hormone. Even if they have too many hormones floating around, their cells no longer accept the hormone or respond to it (Cander, Gul, & Ersoy, 2014). This is often the result of long-term use of high-level hormone replacement therapy. This eventually burns out thyroid production, and disconnects the brain from the thyroid. In this case, the thyroid problem is actually an overmedication problem.

The last common cause of thyroid dysfunction is *autoimmune thyroid disease*, or *Hashimoto's disease*. In this condition, the immune system has been activated against the thyroid gland or against the thyroid peroxidase (TPO) that creates thyroid hormones and is actively attacking and destroying thyroid tissue. Without serious lifestyle intervention, the immune system will eventually destroy the thyroid gland, and the person will have a lifelong dependency upon hormone replacement therapy.

Autoimmune thyroid disease is the most common form of true hypothyroidism in the United States (Zaletel & Gaberšček, 2011). It is rarely tested for and often misdiagnosed as depression (Ayhan et al., 2014) or an anxiety disorder (Carta et al., 2004). And if it is properly diagnosed, it is poorly understood and completely mismanaged.

I say this because the autoimmune thyroid patient is given the exact same hormone treatment as everyone else. Nothing is done to support the immune system. The message that is sent to the autoimmune patient is that there is nothing that can be done to help them, their thyroid gland will eventually be destroyed, so they might as well go on hormones now, because they will be using them for the rest of their life. In this case, the thyroid problem is actually an immune system problem.

I just can't emphasize enough how important it is to have a proper understanding of the autoimmune aspect of many health problems. In fact, 20 percent of the U.S. population (50 million people) currently suffers from some form of autoimmunity. Many of these individuals don't even know they have an autoimmune condition, and those who do are often not being offered any lasting help.

Blood Tests for Thyroid Hormones

Considering the incredible complexity of thyroid function, you must have the correct testing to identify where things might not be working properly. It's not enough to just look at TSH. In fact, many thyroid problems exist within a normal TSH range. T4 is also not enough. Unfortunately, though, this is where testing ends in most medical clinics. You need to also look at T3, to see if thyroid hormones are being converted properly. If there is a suspicion of a conversion problem, then an evaluation of liver and digestive function is warranted.

You need to look at reverse T3, to see if too many hormones are converting into an unusable form of T3. Then you also need to look at free T3 and free T4, to see if the hormones are unbound and available to be used. T3 uptake will give you an indirect measure of thyroid-binding globulins to see if hormones are being released properly. If T3 uptake is out of range, you may then want to follow up with an evaluation of sex hormones to see if there is an estrogen dominance.

Additionally, if TSH is normal or in a low-normal level and you still have hypothyroid symptoms, hypothalamic-pituitary-adrenal axis dysfunction may be suspected, so an evaluation of adrenal function may be appropriate. But please keep in mind that thyroid hormone replacement will artificially lower TSH values, so all results should be considered within the context of current medication use.

Last, every thyroid patient should be tested for thyroglobulin antibodies and TPO antibodies to determine if autoimmunity is involved. If it is, then additional testing for digestive health should be performed.

This is a very important and misunderstood aspect of autoimmunity, so let me explain why I follow up with an evaluation of digestion. Our digestive lining acts as a barrier that protects our insides from the outside. Our immune system patrols the walls looking for invaders and then attacks and destroys them, hopefully before they can invade our bodies and make us sick.

This function is so important that 70 percent of our immune system resides in our digestive tract. As we eat food, our digestive system breaks it down into individual nutrients, and then absorbs it through our digestive lining into our bloodstream to be utilized for energy. If we suffer any damage to the gut's protective lining, it can create a condition known as leaky gut, or intestinal permeability, where partially digested bits of food and other foreign matter or invading antigens are able to leak through into our bloodstream.

This causes our immune system to become overactive as it scrambles to clean up the mess, which further creates a cycle of inflammation and destruction in our digestive tract, until eventually the immune system becomes so overworked that it targets some of our own tissue. An unhealthy digestive environment has just triggered autoimmunity.

Recent research indicates that intestinal permeability, or leaky gut, is the underlying cause of most autoimmune conditions (Fasano, 2012). But let's take it one step further and look at some of the common causes of leaky gut and intestinal permeability: inflammation from food sensitivities, chronic high levels of cortisol, poor blood sugar health, frequent use of antibiotics that destroy healthy bacteria, medication use, and environmental exposure to chemicals. And these are all things that are a common part of the American lifestyle.

Is it starting to make sense, now, why autoimmunity is becoming more and more common in the United States?

CONVENTIONAL VERSUS FUNCTIONAL APPROACHES TO SUPPORTING THYROID HEALTH

Let's discuss the difference between a conventional medical approach for managing thyroid symptoms and the functional wellness and lifestyle approach to supporting thyroid hormone health.

What Is the Conventional Approach?

In a typical medical office, your doctor will perform the blood test for TSH. If it is high, the assumption is that the reason your brain is sending out a lot of TSH to signal the thyroid gland is because the gland is not producing enough thyroid hormone. Thyroid hormone replacement is then prescribed.

A conventional approach might take treatment a step further and test your levels of T3 and T4. But either way, the most common hormone that's going to be prescribed is a synthetic form of T4 called synthroid or levothyroxine. If your doctor checked T3 levels, they might also prescribe a synthetic T3, such as Cytomel or liothyronine. Six weeks later, TSH is checked again, and if it has come down into a normal range, you are considered fixed and you will be checked periodically to make adjustments to your dose. Unfortunately, this sort of protocol is only effective for treating primary hypothyroidism, as I mention earlier. Yet, this is the recommendation that is given for *every* form of hypothyroidism.

If your doctor does check T4 and, in rare cases, T3, then they might decide to provide you with another form of formal treatment, called *bioidentical hormones* or *Armour thyroid*. Armour thyroid provides both T3 and T4. This may be more effective for some people, especially if thyroid conversion is a problem, because it provides the body with some amount of that end product, T3 (Hoang et al., 2013). However, this treatment is still just a Band-Aid for the problem, albeit a better Band-Aid. In most cases, though, it is not enough to simply focus on thyroid hormone levels. Successful management requires addressing the other organ systems that are involved.

An "Inspire Wellness" Experience

Wendy finally got answers about her underlying thyroid problem and was shown a personalized lifestyle program to feel better. Her husband supported her through the process:

"This has been lifesaving for both of us. Together we have lost 89 pounds in 3 months, which is a huge success. I have nothing but great things to say about Dr. Botts and his team. I would highly recommend anybody to come and just sit down and talk with him, because your life will be changed forever."

~ Wendy B.
Round Rock, Texas

What Is the Functional Approach?

The functional approach to support thyroid health involves addressing the organ systems that are involved and have become dysfunctional. Let's go through the causes of hypothyroid symptoms that we discussed earlier and briefly review the functional approach to dealing with them.

First, if the hypothalamic-pituitary-adrenal axis is involved—meaning, for example, if you see normal or low TSH and you see normal or low thyroid hormones — then the adrenal glands are likely involved. That means that an adrenal repair program would be appropriate, which we discussed in an earlier chapter. You need to work on reestablishing communication between the adrenals and the brain. This ultimately requires applying the principles behind both the insulin and the adrenal chapters of this book, since blood sugar health is also closely tied in with adrenal health.

If hormone conversion is the problem, then the liver and digestive system need to be supported. A good liver detox protocol can yield great results for thyroid hormone conversion. This is just one more reason why all of our new practice members at the Inspire Wellness Center start their program with my liver detox and digestive repair protocol.

If thyroid-binding globulins are the problem, then supporting estrogen and other sex hormones is key. You can refer to the previous chapter on estrogen and sex hormones for the principles behind supporting that aspect of health.

Thyroid Resistance

Thyroid resistance is a tough one, because this individual has likely been on thyroid hormone replacement for years, or even decades. About a year ago, I consulted with a new client, and she told me that she had been taking thyroid hormones for *forty years*. It was only after going through comprehensive testing that we identified the underlying reason why she had suffered from this thyroid dysfunction for so long: the source was, in fact, autoimmunity.

As you can imagine, though, she likely had thyroid resistance from burning out the thyroid, or causing the cells to become less receptive to hormones due to four decades of replacement therapy. Unfortunately, these people will often end up depending on lifelong hormone treatment.

However, there is still hope.

By addressing all of the other areas of the body through a holistic approach, I have seen some clients become able to work with their physician on slowly reducing their medication needs. This must always be a slow process, because the body has become dependent upon external thyroid hormone supplementation.

Think about it, though: Why would your thyroid gland keep working to produce something that it's getting elsewhere for free?

Autoimmune Thyroid

First off, let me make one thing very clear. As of right now, there is no medical cure for autoimmune diseases of any form. Once triggered, it is a life sentence. However, that does not mean that you have to sit around doing nothing, waiting for your thyroid gland to be destroyed. Through the proper application of lifestyle modification, many individuals are able to support their immune systems, prevent or slow down thyroid gland destruction, and increase healthy, natural hormone production, which then ultimately improves their symptoms and quality of life.

The functional wellness approach to supporting autoimmune thyroid revolves around first identifying and addressing the triggers of leaky gut, and eliminating or reducing them. Blood tests for immune reactions to foods can determine whether wheat, gluten,[1] dairy, rice, corn, and many other foods are causing inflammation and destruction to the digestive lining. If so, these foods must be strictly avoided.

---

1 Gluten-free diets are not a fad. Even in nonceliac individuals, gluten has the ability to plug into receptors on our intestinal cells, creating leaky gut. Additionally, gluten looks almost identical to thyroid tissue, so if your immune system is attacking the thyroid, there is a high probability that it will attack gluten as well. This can cause a vicious cycle of gluten exposure, immune activation, and then thyroid destruction. For these reasons, I always recommend a gluten-free diet to autoimmune thyroid clients, as well as avoiding any other foods that test reactive on advanced blood testing.

First, I would like to clarify what I mean by immune-reactive foods. This is not the same thing as a food allergy. Many individuals who suspect food sensitivities are tested for food allergies and are told they are not sensitive to anything. However, advanced blood tests reveal a severe immune reaction to some of their favorite foods.

How is this possible?

The short answer: allergic (or anaphylactic) reactions are mediated by a completely different branch of the immune system, compared to delayed sensitivity reactions that occur in the gut. This is why correct testing by a skilled practitioner is key.

In addition to proper food elimination, supplementation of healthy oils, digestive enzymes, probiotics, fermented foods, and herbal compounds can support digestive repair. In some cases, with proper support, the body can heal itself of leaky gut. In more severe cases, though, some diet modifications need to be lifelong.

If symptoms of acid reflux accompany digestive dysfunction, then adding a supplement of hydrochloric acid or vinegar products can help increase stomach acid levels to help improve the breakdown of food, and reduce those reflux symptoms. If cortisol is the suspected trigger and adrenal dysfunction is identified, then an adrenal repair program is appropriate. Other targeted vitamins, minerals, and herbs to support thyroid hormone production and conversion, and to prevent oxidative stress and destruction, can also help. These recommendations should always be tailored to the individual by a qualified healthcare professional who has performed proper lab testing to determine the need. Please, do not accept a one-size-fits-all approach.

Treating the Body as a Whole

Hopefully, by now, you see that thyroid dysfunction is a whole-body problem, and requires a whole-body solution. Let's review the organ systems that must work together in order to achieve proper thyroid balance.

First, the brain, especially the hypothalamus and pituitary glands, are needed in order to activate the thyroid gland. Second, the thyroid gland itself needs to be able to produce adequate levels of hormones. Third, the liver and digestive system need to be able to convert the inactive T4 into the active T3. Sex hormones need to be balanced, but estrogen especially, to prevent an increase in thyroid-binding globulins. Next, blood sugar needs to be controlled to prevent sex hormone imbalance or adrenal dysfunction. And the adrenal glands need to provide appropriate feedback to the brain to balance hypothalamus and pituitary gland output, bringing us full circle to thyroid gland stimulation by the hypothalamus and pituitary gland.

I would never expect to teach someone complete self-management of thyroid health in just one chapter. But hopefully this information has at least given you an overview of why so many people continue to struggle with thyroid symptoms, when all they're doing is taking thyroid hormones. Hopefully, this information can help empower you to start to seek out the solution that's going to fit and that's going to be individualized for you.

Conclusion

At this point, my hope and intention is that this book has offered a clear explanation regarding why our country seems to be getting sicker with each passing year, and how our current healthcare system fails to address this problem. I've covered some of the common hormonal imbalances that result as our body fails to adapt to environmental stressors, creating a state of dis-ease that, if not addressed through proper lifestyle changes, leads to many of the chronic diseases that plague our country. Last, I've given you a brief introduction to the world of functional wellness, and how it offers nutrition, education, and lifestyle solutions that can help us take control of our health. There is better health awaiting all of us if we will learn why things haven't been working up until this point and then choose to start down a different path toward healing.

As a summary, let's cover what this path looks like. There are eight steps to functional wellness that I believe each of us must fulfill in order to achieve our health goals. These are the same eight steps that I use with all of our members at the Inspire Wellness Center.

1. Order the correct test. Far too many people give up after they are told there is nothing wrong, that it's all in their head, or that there's nothing

that can be done to help them. Remember: just because traditional lab tests may say something is normal doesn't mean that it is normal for you. Just because traditional medicine says that there isn't anything that can be done to help you doesn't mean that you can't be doing something to help yourself. If your body is telling you that something is wrong, *trust it*. Don't give up until you find someone who will dig deeper and order the correct test to give you answers.

2. Determine the true underlying cause of dysfunction.

   Always ask the question, "Why?"

   If a lab says your cholesterol or blood sugar is high, or your thyroid hormones are low, don't stop there. Dig deeper to find out why your body is deviating from optimal health and function.

3. Focus on the cause, not the symptom.

   If your blood pressure is high and you take a blood pressure medication to lower it, have you fixed the problem?

   No. You've simply masked it or covered it up. High blood sugar, cholesterol, blood pressure, and hormone changes — these are all symptoms of poor health, not the cause. If all you do is take the pills, without doing anything to support the body's innate ability to heal, then if you ever remove the pills you can expect all the old problems to return. In fact, they've been there the whole time, just hiding and waiting for you to slowly ride down the conveyor belt to poor health.

4. Correct the dysfunction; don't simply alter your labs with drugs. Pills and medications will make things look better. Heck, they will probably even make you feel better, at least for a while. But the true cause of most chronic disease is lifestyle, and there is no pill or medication for lifestyle.

5. Address the body as a whole. I cannot stress this enough. Don't think of yourself as one sick organ, or one imbalanced hormone. Everything must be addressed together, and everything must work together.

6. Have a proven system to follow. Ninety-four percent of all failure is due to not having a system. Most of our practice members who ultimately find success with us do so only after they have tried, and tried, and tried, and failed many times on their own. It wasn't for lack of trying or lack of motivation that they failed previously; it was because they were following the wrong path.

What good is putting in all the hard work to climb a mountain if you reach the top and realize that you're on the wrong peak?

7. Have the right mentor to guide you. It's important to have the right support team to ensure your success. Choose as a mentor someone who does what you want to do, follows the lifestyle that you want to follow, and has achieved the level of health that you want for yourself and your family.

   This is what I call "being in the trenches" with you.

8. Have the right purpose. Any time I sit down for a consultation with a new member at the Inspire Wellness Center, there are a few questions that I ask to help the person put into perspective how their health has been affecting their life and relationships.

   After we've reviewed their health history and concerns, and their prior labs and treatments, I always ask, "Imagine that nothing changes, and you just keep following the path that you are currently on. Where do you see yourself in three to five years?"

   You would be shocked by some of the sobering answers that I've heard to that question:

"Fatter." "Sicker." "More depressed." "In a nursing home." "Dead."

I then ask, "How would your health be different in three to five years if you could resolve your health concerns?"

Finally I ask, "Are you prepared to make the appropriate lifestyle changes that may be necessary in order to achieve your health goals?"Now, fellow reader—and traveler down this path toward health—let me ask you: What are you not happy about with your health?

Why is it that what you're doing right now is not working?

Where do you think your current approach will take you?

Where do you want to be instead?

Are you ready to make the changes and do what will be required to get there?

Do you have the right help to get you from where you are to where you want to go?

If what I've shared with you makes sense, then I'd like to now invite you to put this book down and start to take action. It is true that procrastination is the killer of our health. The last thing I would want is for you to read this book, feel like you've learned some valuable information, but ultimately not be able to take any steps to apply this information to the benefit of your own well-being.

I do a lot of public speaking and people often approach me after the talk and thank me for the information and the presentation.

They'll tell me, "Boy, Dr. Botts, this was wonderful! You sure gave me a lot to go home and think about."

I always wonder where that person is six months later, because I certainly don't see most of these people again. I imagine that they are probably still at home thinking about it, and haven't actually done anything to make themselves feel any better. I feel that I've probably failed that person if they haven't been able to actually change anything based on what they've learned.

I want to give you an opportunity to *not* participate in the "think about it" program, because the results will be to remain exactly where you are right now. We've now spent some time getting to know each other through this book; I'd like to invite you to come in and sit down with me for a one-on-one consultation, so that we can discuss your healthcare needs and start to individualize your plan of action.

We have a special offer for anyone who has read this book. If you would like to know more about this offer, you can call our office or visit our website and we'll be happy to guide you to take the first step toward reclaiming your health.

Next Steps

If what I've shared with you in this book makes sense, if it rings true, then I want to encourage you to start taking steps to make positive changes for your health. At the Inspire Wellness Center, we offer individualized lifestyle programs that include a comprehensive level of evaluation, laboratory testing and analysis, nutrition and exercise counseling, and health education.

If you are in the Austin, Texas, area, please call our office at 512-592-0768 to receive a special offer for an initial wellness consultation. You can also contact us through our website at www.InspireAustin.com. There you will find additional educational material and videos with inspiring stores from our practice. We also offer remote consultations via phone and video chat.

References

Alonso-Magdalena, P., Morimoto, S., Ripoli, C., Fuentes, E., & Nadal, A. (2006). The estrogenic effect of bisphenol A disrupts pancreatic ß-cell function in vivo and induces insulin resistance. *Environmental Health Perspectives,* 106–112.

Ambrosi, B., Masserini, B., Iorio, L., Delnevo, A., Malavazos, A. E., Morricone, L, Sburlai, L. F., & Orsi, E. (2010). Relationship of thyroid function with body mass index and insulin-resistance in euthyroid obese subjects. *Journal of Endocrinological Investigation, 33,* 9, 640–643.

Ayhan, M. G., Uguz, F., Askin, R., & Gonen, M. S. (2014). The prevalence of depression and anxiety disorders in patients with euthyroid Hashimoto's thyroiditis: A comparative study. *General Hospital Psychiatry, 36,* 1, 95–98.

Brand, J. S., Van Der Tweel, I., Grobbee, D. E., Emmelot-Vonk, M. H., & Van Der Schouw, Y. T. (2011). Testosterone, sex hormone-binding globulin and the metabolic syndrome: A systematic review and meta-analysis of observational studies. *International Journal of Epidemiology, 40,* 1, 189–207.

Cander, S., Gul, O. O., & Ersoy, C. (2014). Atypical thyroid function tests, thyroid hormone resistance (Atipik tiroid fonsiyon testleri: Tiroid Hormon Direnci). *Medicine Science/International Medical Journal, 3,* 1545–1570. In Turkish. doi:10.5455/medscience.2014.03.8137.

Carta, M. G., Loviselli, A., Hardoy, M. C., Massa, S., Cadeddu, M., Sardu, C., Carpiniello, B., Dell/Osso, L., & Mariotti, S. (2004). The link between thyroid autoimmunity (antithyroid peroxidase autoantibodies) with anxiety and mood disorders in the community: A field of interest for public health in the future. *BMC Psychiatry, 4,* 1, 25.

Centers for Disease Control and Prevention (2014). National diabetes statistics report: estimates of diabetes and its burden in the United States, 2014. (Atlanta, GA: U.S. Department of Health and Human Services).

Cherry, N., Moore, H., McNamee, R., Pacey, A., Burgess, G., Clyma, J.-A., Dippnall, M., Baillie, H., & Povey, A. (2008). Occupation and male infertility: Glycol ethers and other exposures. *Occupational and Environmental Medicine, 65,* 10, 708–714.

Choi, H., Schmidbauer, N., Sundell, J., Hasselgren, M., Spengler, J., & Bornehag, C.-G. (2010). Common household chemicals and the allergy risks in pre-school age children. *PLOS One, 5,* 10, e13423. doi:10.1371/journal.pone.0013423.

Elbert, E. C. (2010). The thyroid and the gut. *Journal of Clinical Gastroenterology, 44,* 6, 402–406.

Express (2015, September 27). Statins: Heart disease drug speeds up ageing process, warns new research. Accessed at http://www.express.co.uk/life-style/health/608210/statins-age-you-faster-new-research-suggests-long-term-use-warning.

Fasano, A. (2012). Leaky gut and autoimmune diseases. *Clinical Reviews in Allergy & Immunology, 42,* 1, 71–78.

Garduño-Garcia, J. de Jesus, Alvirde-Garcia, U., López-Carrasco, G., Mendoza, M. E. P., Mehta, R., Arellano-Campos, O., Choza, R., et al. (2010). TSH and free thyroxine concentrations are associated with differing metabolic markers in euthryroid subjects. *European Journal of Endocrinology, 163,* 2, 273–278.

Garlin, M. C., Arnold, A. M., Lee, J. S., Robbins, J., & Cappola, A. R. (2014). Subclinical Dysfunction and Hip Fracture and Bone mineral density in older adults: The cardiovascular health study. doi:http://dx.doi.org/10.1210/jc.2014-1951. Accessed at http://press.endocrine.org/doi/abs/10.1210/jc.2014-1051.

Grossman, M., Thomas, M. C., Panagiotopoulos, S., Sharpe, K., MacIsaac, R. J., Clarke, S., Zajac, J. D., & Jerums, G. (2013). Low testosterone levels are common and associated with insulin resistance in men with diabetes. *Journal of Clinical Endocrinology & Metabolism, 93,* 1834–1840.

Harvey, P. W., & Darbre, P. (2004). Endocrine disrupters and human health: Could oestrogenic chemicals in body care cosmetics adversely affect breast cancer incidence in women? *Journal of Applied Toxicology, 24,* 3, 167–176.

Hayes, T. B., Anderson, L. L., Beasley, V. R., de Solla, S. R., Iguchi, T., Ingraham, H., Kesteomnt, P., et al. (2011). Demasculinization and feminization of male gonads by atrazine: Consistent effects across vertebrate classes. *The Journal of Steroid Biochemistry and Molecular Biology, 127,* 1, 64–73.

Healthline (2014, September 8). Type 2 diabetes statistics and facts. Accessed at: http://www.healthline.com/health/type-2-diabetes/statistics#2

Hoang, T. D. Olsen, C. H., Mai, V. Q., Clyde, P. W., & Shakir, M. K. M. (2013). Dessicated thyroid extract compared with levothyroxine in the treatment of hypothyroidism: A randomized, double-blind, crossover study. *Journal of Clinical Endocrinolgy & Metabolism, 98,* 5, 1982–1990.

Jaga, K., & Dharmani, C. (2003). Sources of exposure to and public health implications of organophosphate pesticides. *Revista panamericana de salud pública, 14,* 3, 171–185.

Kalra, S., Gopalakrishnan, A., Unnikrishnan, A. G., & Sahay, R. (2014). The hypoglycemic side of hypothyroidism. *Indian Journal of Endocrinology and Metabolism, 18,* 1, 1.

Kessler, H., Sisson, S., & Short, K. Potential for high-intensity interval training to reduce cardiometabolic disease risk. (2012, June 1). *SportsMed, 42,* 6, 489–509.

Lovallo, W., et al. Caffeine stimulation of cortisol secretion across the waking hours in relation to caffeine intake levels (2005). *Psychosom. Med., 67,* 5, 734–739. doi:10.1097/01.psy. oooo181270.20036.06.

Lacasaña, M. et al. (2010). Association between organophosphate pesticides exposure and thyroid hormones in floriculture workers. *Toxicology and Applied Pharmacology, 243,* 1, 19–26.

Nussey, S., & Whitehead, S. A. (2001). The thyroid gland. In *Endocrinology: An Integrated Approach.* Oxford, UK: Bios. Retrieved from www.ncbi. nlm.nih.gov/books/NBK28/.

Nygaard, B. (2016). Hypothyroidism (primary). Systematic Review 605. *BMJ Clinical Evidence.* Accessed January 14 from http://clinicalevidence.bmj.com/x/systematic-review/0605/overview.html.

Pflieger-Bruss, S., Schuppe, H.-C., & Schill, W.-B. (2004). The male reproductive system and its susceptibility to endocrine disrupting chemicals. *Andrologia, 36,* 6, 337–345.

Santin, A. P., & Furlanetto, T. W. (2011, May 4). Role of estrogen in thyroid function and growth regulation. *Journal of Thyroid Research.* Retrieved from http://www.ncbi.nlm.nih.gov/pmc/articles/PMC3113168/.

Sheehan, M. T. (2004). Polycystic ovarian syndrome: Diagnosis and management. *Clinical Medicine & Research, 2,* 1, 13–27.

Shin, D.-J., & Osborne, T. F. (2004). Thyroid hormone regulation and cholesterol metabolism are connected through sterol regulatory element-binding protein-2 (SREBP-2). *Journal of Biological Chemistry, 278,* 36, 34114–34118.

Suba, Z. (2012). Interplay between insulin resistance and estrogen deficiency as co-activators in carcinogenesis. *Pathology & Oncology Research, 18,* 2, 123–133.

Talbott, S. M. (2007). *The cortisol connection: Why stress makes you fat and ruins your health – and what you can do about it.* Alameda, CA: Hunter House.

Tjønna, A. et al. (2008). Aerobic interval training versus continuous moderate exercise as a treatment for the metabolic syndrome: A pilot study. *Circulation, 118,* 4, 346–354.

U.S. Food and Drug Administration (U.S. FDA) (2014). FDA expands advice on statin risks. *FDA Consumer Health Information.* http://www.fda.gov/downloads/ForConsumers/ConsumerUpdates/UCM293705.htm.

Völzke, H., Robinson, D. M., & John, U. (2005). Association between thyroid function and gallstone disease. *World Journal of Gastroenterology, 11,* 35, 5530–5534.

World Health Organization (WHO) (2015). Global Health Observatory Data Repository: Life Expectancy — Data by Country (CSV). Geneva, Switzerland: World Health Statistics.

Zaletel, K., & Gaberšžek, S. (2011). Hashimoto's thyroiditis: From genes to the disease. *Current Genomics, 12,* 8, 576.

About the Author

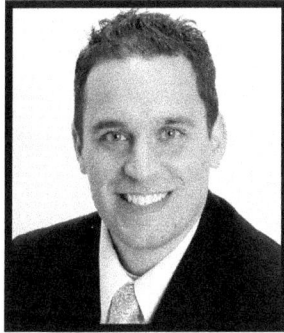

Dr. Trevor Botts is a wellness expert on lifelong optimized living. His passion for healthy living and dedication to helping others reach their health goals has resulted in a breakthrough lifestyle program, proving that health and vitality can be reclaimed by just about any proactive person at any age.

Dr. Botts is an engaging public speaker who has educated thousands through his health seminars, corporate workshops, and private classes. He has been featured on NBC and CBS as an advocate for restoring true prevention to healthcare, offering natural, noninvasive programs for gaining and preserving wellness through broad lifestyle enrichment rather than disease management. His professional education includes doctor of chiropractic, functional wellness, nutrition, and fitness. He is also president and clinical director of the Inspire Wellness Center.

Dr. Botts lives in Austin, Texas, with his wife, Amanda, and their three children, Elijah, Jocelyn and Logan.

www.ingramcontent.com/pod-product-compliance
Lightning Source LLC
Chambersburg PA
CBHW071223290326
41931CB00037B/1952